Conquer Your Emetophobia

also by this author

Emetophobia

Understanding and Treating Fear of Vomiting in Children and Adults

Dr David Russ and Anna S. Christie

Foreword by Dr David Veale

ISBN 978 1 83997 657 5
eISBN 978 1 83997 658 2

of related interest

Free Yourself from Emetophobia

A CBT Self-Help Guide for a Fear of Vomiting

Alexandra Keyes and David Veale

ISBN 978 1 78775 331 0
eISBN 978 1 78775 332 7

Your Worry Makes Sense

Anxiety and Burnout Are Logical (and You Can Overcome Them)

Dr Martin Brunet

Illustrated by Hannah Robinson

ISBN 978 1 80501 297 9
eISBN 978 1 80501 298 6
Audio ISBN 978 1 39982 756 0

The OCD Recovery Journal

Creative Activities to Keep Yourself Well

Cara Lisette and Phoebe Webb

Foreword by Ashley Fulwood

Illustrated by Victoria Barron

ISBN 978 1 80501 095 1
eISBN 978 1 80501 096 8

20 Ways to Break Free from Trauma

From Brain Hijacking to Post-Traumatic Growth

Philippa Smethurst

Foreword by Sir Terry Waite

ISBN 978 1 80501 310 5
eISBN 978 1 80501 311 2

CONQUER YOUR EMETOPHOBIA

Advice from a Therapist Who Overcame the Fear of Vomiting

Anna S. Christie

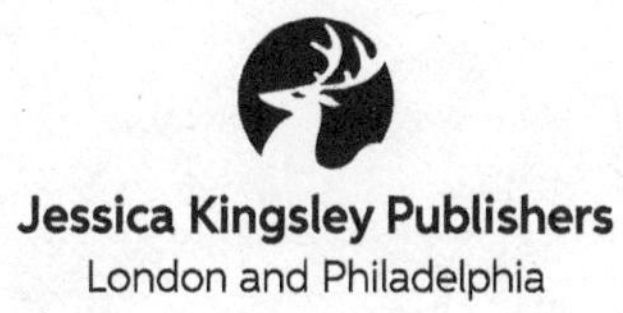

Jessica Kingsley Publishers
London and Philadelphia

First published in Great Britain in 2026 by Jessica Kingsley Publishers
An imprint of John Murray Press

1

The information contained in this book is not intended to replace the services of trained medical professionals or to be a substitute for medical advice. You are advised to consult a doctor on any matters relating to your health, and in particular on any matters that may require diagnosis or medical attention.

A CIP catalogue record for this title is available from the
British Library and the Library of Congress

ISBN 978 1 80501 776 9
eISBN 978 1 80501 777 6

Printed and bound in the United States by Integrated Books International

Jessica Kingsley Publishers' policy is to use papers that are natural, renewable and recyclable products and made from wood grown in sustainable forests. The logging and manufacturing processes are expected to conform to the environmental regulations of the country of origin.

Jessica Kingsley Publishers
Carmelite House
50 Victoria Embankment
London EC4Y 0DZ

www.jkp.com

John Murray Press
Part of Hodder & Stoughton Ltd
An Hachette Company

The authorised representative in the EEA is Hachette Ireland,
8 Castlecourt Centre, Dublin 15, D15 XTP3, Ireland (email: info@hbgi.ie)

For Sheila.

Acknowledgments

I would first like to acknowledge and thank Editor Jane Evans of Jessica Kingsley Publishers for inviting me to write this book as "part self-help and part memoir." It has been an enriching experience working with JKP again. I thank all the people along the way who helped me or simply put up with me during my 25-year healing journey. My mother, for teaching me that tummies have all sorts of non-worrisome troubles; my husband, for enduring me and my phobia at its worst; my three kids whom I love more than life itself; my grandkids, for giving me a second chance at treating a vomiting child "normally;" my wonderful psychologist, Dr. Geoffrey Carr, who facilitated my healing from trauma and helped me become a better human being and one who could experience joy in all circumstances of life. And finally, my beautiful sister, Sheila, to whom this book is dedicated, who lifted me up out of physical disability and despair by simply walking with me every day for two years, when at first I could only make it as far as the neighbor's car. Without her selfless and thoughtful actions, I would never have had the energy to write this book or participate in many of the other wonderful activities I can now enjoy.

Contents

Contents

Introduction

WHAT IS EMETOPHOBIA?

Emetophobia is an irrational yet very severe fear of...let's call it *the thing* for now. You know what I'm talking about, but you may be terrified at this point to even see the word in print. I understand that if you have just picked up this book and taken a gingerly peek at the first page, you may also have been afraid of seeing any other word that refers to *the thing*. I will try to ease you into it as slowly and as gently as possible.

The thing starts with the letter "v," and for many people with emetophobia, hearing the word, or seeing it written, sends them into a spiral of panic. If you do not have emetophobia and you are reading this book to try to understand more about it, you may think I'm being ridiculous, but check out emetophobia groups on social media. All but one (my group, which I named "Emetophobia No Panic") asks people to abbreviate *the thing* by using just the letter "v" followed by an asterisk. And it doesn't stop there. The feeling you get right before *the thing* happens? That's abbreviated as "n*," as are a plethora of other words related to *the thing*. It may seem strange to people who don't have emetophobia, but I believe, rather, that it is indicative of just how frightening *the thing* is to people who do.

I had very severe emetophobia for two-thirds of my life. If I saw the word in a book or magazine, I would burst into tears and it would ruin my entire day. The thoughts would continue to swirl around in my mind, haunting me, *jinxing me*, as I believed at the time. Today, as I write this, I am completely phobia-free. I now make my living helping other people who are afraid of *the thing*—as a licensed therapist I've treated over 300 patients with emetophobia. I teach classes, host a podcast, and talk to thousands of people with emetophobia online. Yet outside of work I never even think about *the thing*.

The small amount of research into emetophobia has shown that 7 percent of people are afraid of *the thing*; about 0.2 percent are so afraid that they will seek treatment for it.[1] This means that at least 16 million people worldwide have diagnosable emetophobia. It is therefore a very common phobia, yet most people who have it are so humiliated that they hide it from everyone.

Sometimes, folks react to you telling them about this phobia with silly responses such as, "Well, nobody likes it." As if you never thought of that. As if you're someone who is exactly like everyone else who doesn't like it, except that you are a drama queen who revels in negative attention or is just plain acting insane.

I still witness people responding to me about my work with emetophobia with incredulity. It seems that a fear of heights, small places, clowns, or bees is more socially acceptable than a fear of *the thing*. Perhaps it is the bodily function aspect that makes it more embarrassing, the fact that it is normally done in private and in a washroom.

Some people outright tell us that we're stupid, weak, or insane, and so the phobia remains largely hidden. In the '60s and '70s, when I was growing up, I would never have dared to utter a word about it. News flash: emetophobia is common! And it is one of the most severe and debilitating phobias in existence.

Emetophobia may entail a fear of doing *the thing* yourself, seeing or hearing others do it, or any combination of those. It is listed in the *Diagnostic and Statistical Manual of Mental Disorders* as "specific phobia: other type."[2] *The thing* is listed as an example, along with the fear of choking. To be diagnosed with emetophobia, the fear must prevent you from living life in a typical way, or your response to the feared *thing* must be extreme, or what is often referred to as causing a "full-blown panic attack."

If you've purchased this book, you have probably diagnosed yourself with emetophobia, which is very easy to do. If you're not sure, there is

---

1 Philips, H. C. (1985) "Return of fear in the treatment of a fear of vomiting." *Behavior Research and Therapy* 23, 1, 45–52. https://doi.org/10.1016/0005-7967(85)90141-X; Van Hout, W. J. and Bouman, T. K. (2011) "Clinical features, prevalence and psychiatric complaints in subjects with fear of vomiting." *Clinical Psychology and Psychotherapy* 19, 6, 531–539. https://doi.org/10.1002/cpp.761

2 American Psychiatric Association (2022) *Diagnostic and Statistical Manual of Mental Disorders, Fifth Edition, Text Revision: (DSM-5-TR)*. American Psychiatric Association Press.

a questionnaire you can take in Appendix 1 to determine if your diagnosis is correct. Trigger warning: the word is spelled out throughout this questionnaire.

WHAT CAUSES EMETOPHOBIA?

Trauma

Several factors seem to contribute to a development of emetophobia. Sometimes childhood trauma is notably heinous, such as in the case of child abuse by parents or someone else the patient knew. At other times the trauma is different yet still significant. It may or may not be related to *the thing* itself (such as the child having a particularly tough time with a tummy virus). I have only a hazy recollection of the events of October 17, 1962: disjointed impressions, flashes of scenes, memories of my perpetual happy mood, which was incongruous with that of my parents and my 15-year-old sister. I was just a month shy of my fourth birthday.

My brother, Kenny, 17, had been in a motorbike accident, and he was in hospital in a critical condition with a traumatic brain injury. He was in a coma, being kept alive in an iron lung.

I learned later that my parents told me for three days that Kenny was "sick" in the hospital. I don't suppose I knew much about what "sick" meant. The only reference I had was the time Kenny rocked me so hard on my rocking horse that *the thing* happened and my family referred to it as "being sick." This might have been no big deal if Kenny hadn't died three days later.

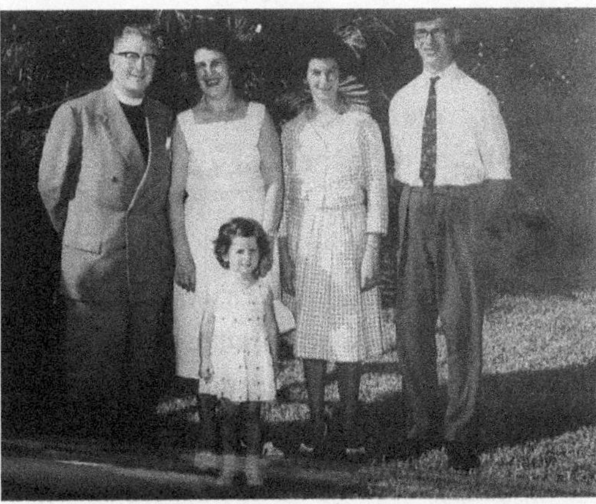

Figure 0.1. The only photograph in existence of my whole family

Although I couldn't put my finger on it until countless hours of therapy later in life, my dad was never the same after Kenny died. That will seem obvious to anyone who has lost a child, but to me, being so young, it was just confusing. My dad had become my pseudo-mom or, as the psychologists now say, "primary attachment figure," when I was just a baby because apparently Mother didn't like children. Whatever the reason, my dad was my everything for as long as I can remember—my #1 person. Mother was just...around.

I now believe that Kenny being "sick" and then dying was the beginning of my phobia. Added to the list of contributing factors may have been the time I swallowed a large Bermuda coin and got it stuck in my throat at age five. A neighbor lady tried to induce *the thing* when that happened by sticking her fingers down my throat and making me drink salt water. Eventually I was taken to hospital and wheeled into surgery, screaming for my dad.

I clung to my dad for several years, until he got colon cancer when I was eight and died just after my ninth birthday. He was sick at home for a long time with *the thing* before he died. My dad's death was the icing on my emetophobia cake.

Other causes

You may not have any traumatic experiences in your memory. Many people have siblings or parents who were ill or died when they were young and they didn't develop emetophobia. So there has to be more to it than that.

There are many misunderstandings and misguided notions about the causes or contributing factors that lead to emetophobia. One is that those who have it must have suffered sexual abuse or assault at some point and may have repressed the memory. In my work with people with emetophobia over the past 20+ years, I have seldom seen this patient history. I have seen a few people who had traumatic childhoods, some of whom experienced sexual abuse or assault, but it is by no means universal, nor even the majority of my patients.

The good news is that it doesn't matter what may have caused or contributed to your emetophobia because the treatment is the same. If you have childhood trauma, I encourage you to work with a therapist toward healing it, although it's not necessary to do that before undergoing treatment for your emetophobia.

Nature or nurture?

One factor that is common among people with emetophobia is that they usually have anxiety, depression, addiction, or abuse somewhere in their family tree. Scientists conclude that a genetic predisposition ("nature") accounts for about 50 percent of a phobia developing. The rest ("nurture") probably comes from some sort of "perfect storm" of emotional experiences in childhood.

The genetic predisposition for anxiety can be carried down through generations, as with descendants of the Holocaust or residential schools in Canada, for example. My mother was incredibly anxious, expressed often in anger, but also in a few phobias of her own.

Your contributing factors

EXERCISE 1: Listing family members

List any family members, going back as many generations as you know of, who had anxiety, depression, addiction, other mental illness or trauma, or even physical illnesses, especially if they were chronic.

....

....

....

....

....

....

....

....

You may not know what happened to you to lead to your emetophobia, or you may have some ideas, or you may think you know for sure, but you could be wrong. For example, I've had patients tell me that they were ill as a child with a virus of some sort, and this is why they have emetophobia. But lots of kids have viruses and were very ill with them as children. One of my grandkids was so ill she was hospitalized twice, but she's not the least bit emetophobic. I would have a total emotional meltdown whenever my kids were ill, but all three of them also escaped emetophobia and so far, every other mental illness. So there is much we do not know.

For some reason I always assumed that I had an okay childhood, and, unbelievably, I thought I didn't experience any trauma. Nobody hit me or sexually assaulted me, and thanks to Mother telling me and everyone else that I didn't remember my brother, I didn't think his death or the series of events that happened subsequently was actually traumatic. I have since spent about 300 hours in therapy exploring my childhood and the impact of its trauma on my life. While this has been very enlightening and helped me grow and change as a person, it didn't make a dent in the phobia's symptoms.

Whether you have trauma or not, it behooves you to have a long talk with your parents and siblings if that is possible. Ask them what may have happened to you before the age of five that you can't necessarily remember now but involved illness of any sort. Because although you may not remember it, *your body remembers it.* Our bodies hold a great deal of anxiety because the part of our brain that warns us of danger records events that happened to us from birth, and some would argue even before birth. What happened to you may be something so minor that you can't even think of it. One of my eight-year-old child patients was ill twice when her mom and dad were away at hospital having babies. Some kids develop anxiety just because mom returns to work or their parents get divorced whereas others seem unaffected by these things.

EXERCISE 2: Recording childhood events

List and/or write about any events that happened to you in your early childhood.

....

....

....

....

....

....

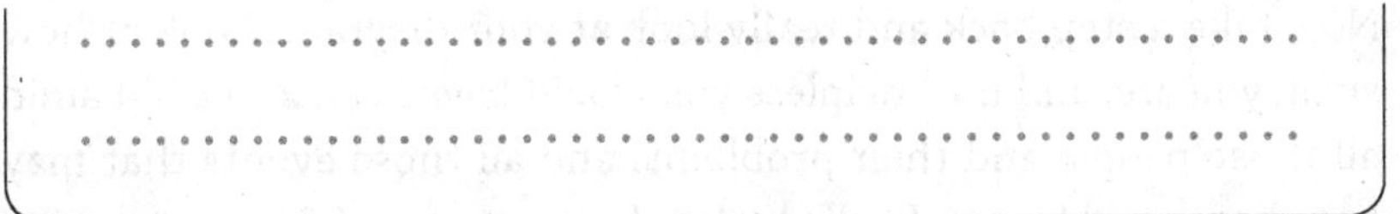

EXERCISE 3: Viewing your contributing factors

Fill in Figure 0.2 with the information from Exercises 1 and 2.

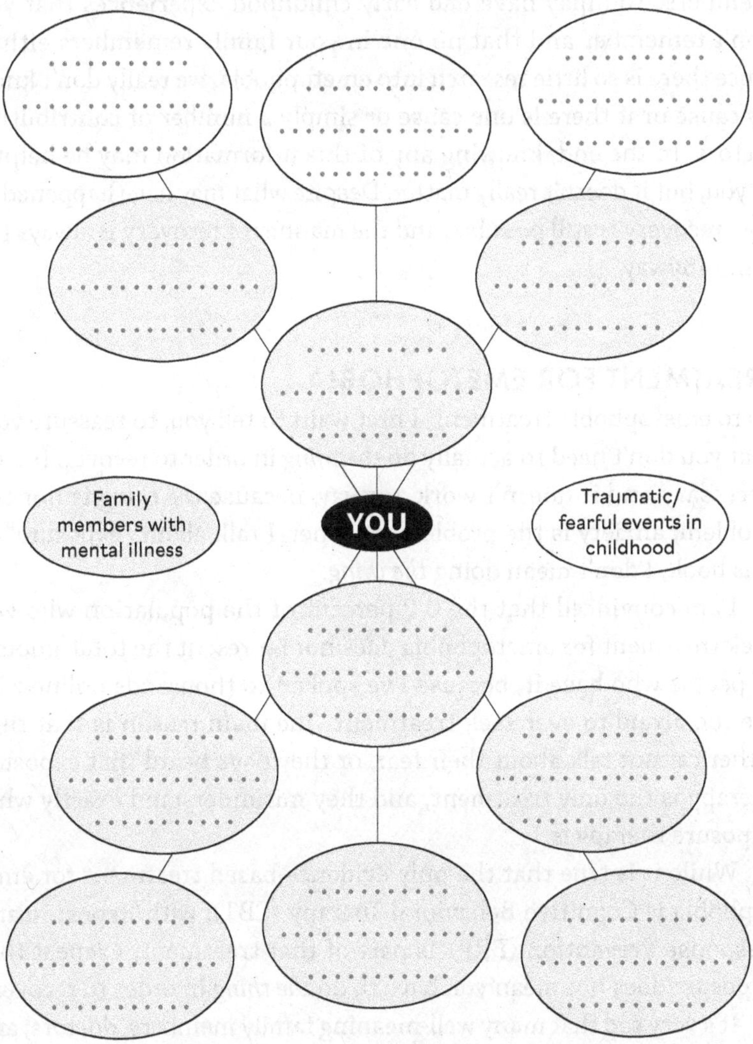

Figure 0.2. Contributing factors to emetophobia

Now take a step back and really look at your diagram. Look at how small you are, and how helpless you would have been as a child amid all those people and their problems, and all those events that may have happened to you. Really look at how out of control you were as a child. But you are not small and helpless now. You still cannot control *the thing*, but you can learn to control your response to it so that it no longer frightens you.

Perhaps you don't know much, or anything, about your family members. You may have had early childhood experiences that you don't remember and that no one in your family remembers either. Since there is so little research into emetophobia, we really don't know its cause or if there is one cause or simply a number of contributing factors. In the end, knowing any of this information may be helpful to you, but it doesn't really matter. Despite what may have happened to you, recovery is still possible, and the manner of recovery is always the same anyway.

TREATMENT FOR EMETOPHOBIA

As to emetophobia treatment, I first want to tell you, to reassure you, that you don't need to actually do *the thing* in order to recover. It isn't necessary and it doesn't work anyway, because *the thing* is not the problem; anxiety is the problem. So when I talk about "exposure" in this book, I don't mean doing *the thing*.

I am convinced that the 0.2 percent of the population who will seek treatment for emetophobia does not represent the total amount of people who have it, because I've spoken to thousands online who are too afraid to ever seek treatment. The main reason is that they either cannot talk about their fear, or they have heard that exposure therapy is the only treatment, and they misunderstand exactly what exposure therapy is.

While it is true that the only evidence-based treatment for emetophobia is Cognitive Behavioral Therapy (CBT), with Exposure and Response Prevention (ERP) as part of that treatment, I repeat that exposure does not mean you have to do *the thing* in order to recover.

It's very sad that many well-meaning family members, doctors, and even therapists suggest to people with emetophobia that they should simply make themselves do *the thing* for their phobia to magically go away. It will not. But the mere suggestion of it may send patients running from the room never to return. Some brave souls have tried inducing *the thing* themselves, and by their own reporting to me or online to other people with emetophobia, it either didn't work, didn't work for long, or made their phobia worse.

People also misunderstand experiences around *the thing* for exposure. For example, many people write in my Facebook group that they had an "exposure" on the weekend because their child was ill. This was not an exposure in the clinical sense of the word; it was an experience and could be one that retraumatized the person. Exposure in the clinical sense is a very gradual and *intentionally constructed* set of experiences beginning with imagination, words, sentences, drawings, pictures of nauseous people, and so on, each going up one baby step, as slowly and cautiously as you are able.

If you think you can't do any exposures, you're wrong—you can. That's because proper exposures start so easily and simply and progress so slowly and gradually that you will only feel some unease or a low level of tolerable distress—never shock, surprise, or horror. Why exposure therapy? Because it is the only evidence-based treatment for emetophobia so far. This means that it is the only method that has been shown in scientific studies to work.

WHAT IF I DO *THE THING* BY CHANCE?

Sometimes people with emetophobia do *the thing* for one reason or another. Usually, right afterward, they feel as if they're not afraid anymore, and this bliss can last for months or even years. For others, it's more of a "honeymoon" of a few days before the phobia returns. Still others are just as afraid afterward as before. Almost exclusively, those who have gone through all the CBT and exposure work have the thought "Hey, it's not that bad" solidified in their brain. It's almost as if all the cognitive work and exposure "clicks into place." This was certainly my experience and that of several others with whom I have worked over the years.

I believe that having an incident of *the thing* with no reference in your brain as to its true meaning (that it isn't dangerous) is what causes the phobia to simply return. To date, only one scientific study[3] has been done on the return of fear to those with this specific phobia.

HOW LONG DOES IT TAKE TO RECOVER?

Although it varies from case to case, it will probably take you at least a year of commitment, self-discipline, and practice. So if you were looking for a quick fix or complete recovery by the time you get to the end of this book, then I'm so sorry for being the one to burst that bubble for you.

I achieved recovery from different aspects of my emetophobia at different times and through different means. It started with a whole focus on eating. A few years later, I participated in a group therapy ERP program, which finally got me over fearing doing *the thing* myself (within about a year), and then over a decade later, I overcame the fear of other people with more ERP that I designed myself. It was another two years before I felt this had worked for me and I was finally over the phobia and living a normal life. My emetophobia recovery journey, in total, took me from 1977 to 2002—about 25 years. So I can't tell you specifically how long it will take you, as someone working on all of it at the same time, but I have seen patients of mine and stories of others who recovered in about a year or two. If you're completely recovered in six months, that will be a nice surprise, and you can come on my podcast and tell us all how you did it.

In this book I will be giving examples from my own life of many of the principles of emetophobia recovery. The examples will not be given in chronological order but rather in the order in which recovery normally takes place. I have provided a list of my experiences in chronological order in Appendix 2, if you are interested.

THE IMPORTANCE OF HOMEWORK

Homework is an integral part of all CBT work. If you are simply seeing your therapist once a week for 50 minutes, even if you are doing exposure exercises, you will be seeing them for years and years if you don't do some homework. Many of my patients and class members

---

3 Philips, H. C. (1985) "Return of fear in the treatment of a fear of vomiting." *Behavior Research and Therapy* 23, 1, 45–52. https://doi.org/10.1016/0005-7967(85)90141-X

ask me how long they should spend doing homework. It's up to the individual, but the more time you spend daily, the quicker you will recover. You should work to accomplish one thing each day, whether you spend 10–15 minutes on it or an hour, although spending an hour is obviously more helpful than spending 10 minutes.

I never ask that people spend more than five days a week on homework. There is no point in replacing your emetophobia with workaholism—just don't get too comfortable. Your brain will convince you that it likes the relaxation better than it likes doing exposure work, and will push you to avoid or procrastinate over the homework.

I beckon you now to come with me on this recovery journey of yours. It won't be that bad and it will ultimately lead you out of your hellish emetophobia life and into a life of peace, joy, and hope.

SUMMARY

- I defined emetophobia as any fear of anything related to *the thing*.
- You may have had trauma in your childhood, as I did, or you may not have.
- You listed any family members with mental or physical disorders ("nature").
- You listed any events that happened in your childhood that may have led to your anxiety ("nurture").
- It doesn't matter what caused your emetophobia because the treatment is the same.
- You don't need to do *the thing* in order to recover from emetophobia.
- "Exposure and Response Prevention therapy," or ERP, may not be what you think it is.
- You can do exposures because they will begin small and easy and progress to more difficult very slowly and gradually.
- Think of your recovery journey in terms of years, not weeks or even months. Many people recover fully in under two years.

Chapter One

GOAL-SETTING

When I had emetophobia there was no help to be found. There wasn't even an internet. No doctors or therapists whom I told about my phobia had ever heard of it before. The therapists who were kind and truly wanted to help often began by asking me the same thing, "What are your goals?" I thought it was a rather silly request at the time. I only had one goal, and that was to not be afraid of *the thing*. A couple of them tried to get me to make a "hierarchy of fears" so that I could face the fears one step at a time. I also didn't understand this request. I was only afraid of seeing or doing *the thing*. Apart from that I wasn't afraid of anything, so I believed there was no hierarchy. I tried several therapists who made similar requests or worse, such as "Go home and drink ipecac so you [do *the thing*]." But that was far too scary for me. It was 10 out of 10 terrifying. The fact that I couldn't do it was the reason I was sitting in their office in the first place.

My patients with emetophobia often tell me the same thing I told my previous therapists, which is that their goal is to "not have emetophobia." I now know it's important with goals to express them in a positive format, rather than beginning with the negative "not." Imagine if someone afraid of dogs, a rather simple specific phobia to treat, said their only goal was not to be afraid of dogs. How would they go about working on that? It seems hopeless by its very nature. However, if their goals were something like "to walk past a leashed dog on a street, to go to a friend's house who owns a nice dog, and to one day pat a dog's head," then you can probably already form a treatment plan for them yourself. Hint: they have to go about doing those things very gradually and at a distance. So let's explore what we need to know to set goals for you before we start any treatment exercises.

In 1981 George T. Doran noticed that many businesses had goals that were too general to be meaningful to them. He wrote that goals must be measurable and, in fact, achievable, in order to move the business forward. He created what is now known by the acronym "SMART" goals. Since his time, business, non-profit organizations, education and the social sciences have embraced SMART goals (Figure 1.1).

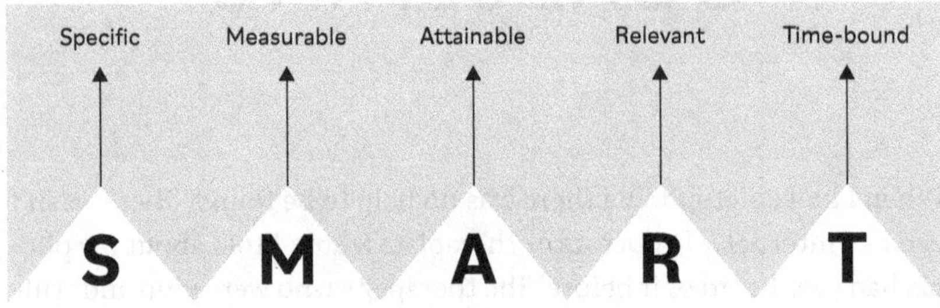

Figure 1.1. SMART goals

SMART GOALS

Specific

I always ask my patients what they would like to do that they feel they can't do now. Setting specific goals also helps me, as their therapist, to know how serious the phobia is. For example, if I'm told that someone's most important goal would be to "leave the house," then I know that patient is far more limited than someone who expresses "flying for travel" as their most important goal. Some other examples of specific goals related to emetophobia might be "staying at a hotel," "cooking chicken properly," or "getting pregnant." If I'd been in treatment for emetophobia when I was younger, my specific goals would have been:

- To visit someone in hospital and stay if I hear or see *the thing*
- To stay upstairs with my kids when they are ill, or even better, to stay with them in the washroom
- To travel on planes, trains, and buses
- To go to a party, or to stay late at a party, when people are drinking too much.

I may have added "To try marijuana or get drunk" back then, but by the time I recovered that ship had pretty much sailed. I don't think I missed much.

In Figure 1.2 list all the things you wish you could do but cannot do now because of your emetophobia.

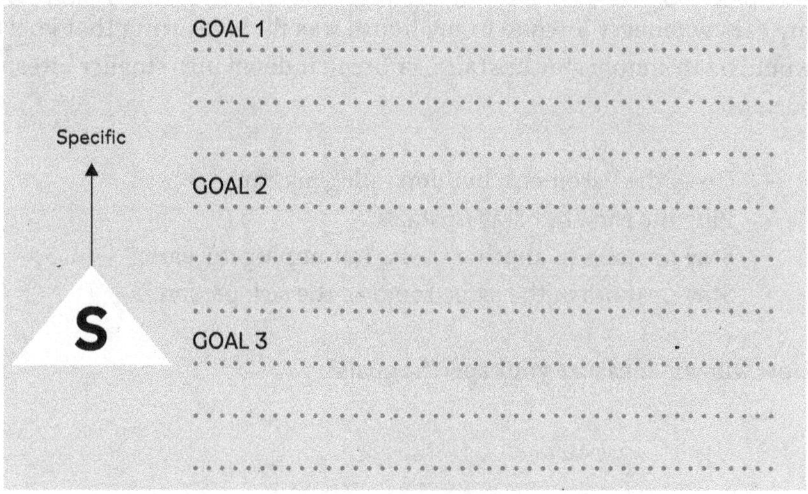

Figure 1.2. Specific

Measurable

With emetophobia, a goal is almost always measurable if it is specific. Goals such as "Be less anxious when my kids are sick" is:

- Expressed in a negative ("be less")
- Not specific, and therefore
- Not measurable.

You may think you will know if you are less anxious, but it's still not very specific. However, the goal of riding in the car around the block with your significant other driving is very specific and therefore measurable.

My most important goal would have been pretty lofty when I was starting exposure therapy. I'd have only had one, and that would have been to stay with someone who was ill and not run down the street screaming and flailing my arms overhead. If I could do that, I figured I would be over the phobia because before doing therapy I was the Usain Bolt of emetophobia. Sometimes I would run away so fast and so instantly that I didn't even know how I got outside into a parking lot. Except I did know, because there was only one thing that sent me running like that. My first career was ministry in the United Church of Canada, which required me to visit the sick in hospital. Let's just say I got to be close friends with all the parking lot attendants. I also got very tired of running down to the basement and plugging my ears whenever anyone in my house was ill. Measuring that goal would be to simply stay upstairs, or break it down into smaller bites, such as:

- Go to the basement, but don't plug my ears.
- Plug my ears, but stay upstairs.
- Stay upstairs in another room, but unplug my ears.
- Stay upstairs in the same room as the sick person.

How will you measure your specific goals?

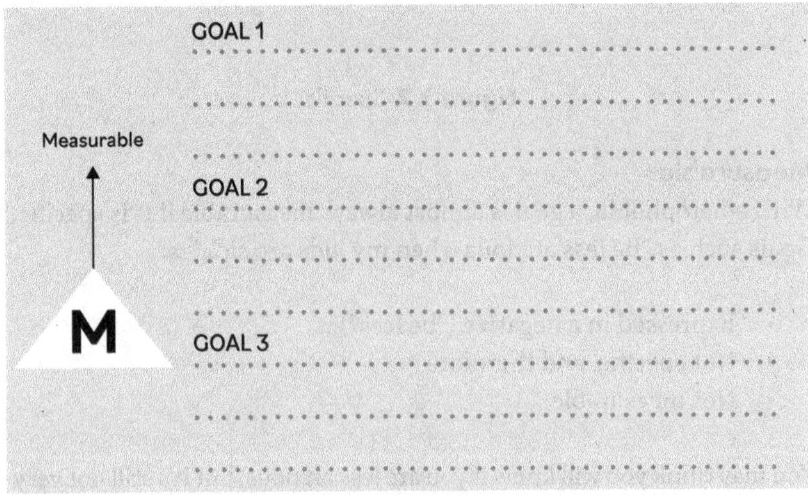

Figure 1.3. Measurable

Attainable

Are your goals realistic? If you can't leave your washroom, have panic attacks all day long, and your average anxiety level is 8 out of 10, it probably isn't attainable to set a goal of flying from Canada to Australia for 19 hours in a few weeks' time. This is an extreme example, but I have found in my clinical practice that many of my patients with emetophobia set goals for themselves that are not really attainable, at least in any given time period. I teach a set of 10 emetophobia recovery classes. Some participants set a goal of being fully recovered at the end of the 10 classes. This is seldom, if ever, attainable.

When I was young I dreamed of becoming a minister like my father. In elementary school I won public speaking contests, and I excelled academically. I knew I had close to eight years of university ahead of me, which would include moving away from home, staying in a dorm with strangers, doing practical courses in hospitals and nursing homes, visiting the sick and elderly, as well as practical work with children in Sunday school, vacation Bible school, and camp. My goal to be a minister was actually unattainable on every level except academics. I decided that in order to pursue this career I must hide my emetophobia and cleverly avoid any situation where someone might do *the thing*. Avoid sick people, old people, and kids. That was my strategy while at the same time constantly looking for help for the emetophobia. While this strategy worked for me in a sense—I became a minister and no one knew about the emetophobia—it was still a life of constant fear, secrecy, and running away. Having a goal that includes avoidance or safety behaviors isn't really a goal; it's just trying to survive without giving anything up.

Are your goals attainable? Explain how in Figure 1.4.

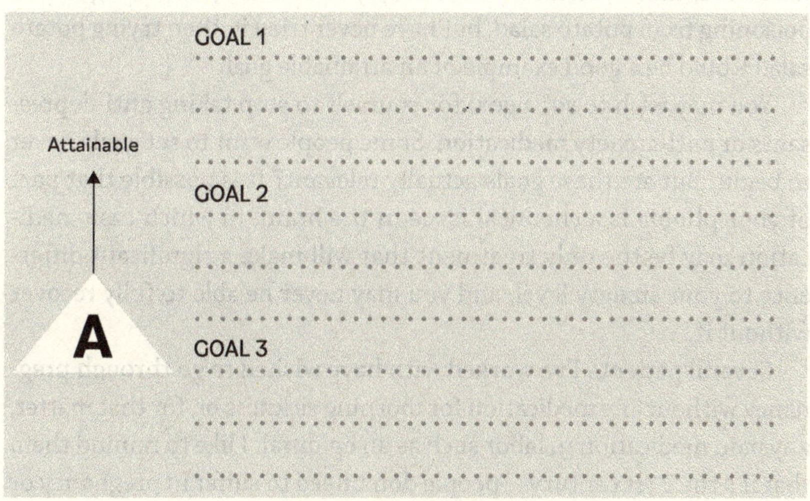

Figure 1.4. Attainable

Relevant

Does your goal contribute to your recovery from emetophobia? The answer to this seems obvious in our context, but I'll share with you some examples of irrelevant goals for people with emetophobia.

My husband doesn't have and never had emetophobia. When he was a teenager, he got drunk on sangria, and it made him very sick (as would any alcohol in excess). Nevertheless, he still blames the sangria itself. So, for the past 50 years, he has turned his nose up at sangria. He doesn't want to look at it or even hear it mentioned. Yet many of my patients set a goal for themselves of eating or drinking something that made them ill at one point in time. There is no point in setting such a goal. Go ahead and avoid sangria or anything else you ate before it made you sick. People without emetophobia do this as a matter of course. I was ill once after eating those pea pods that you stir-fry and I don't ever want to see one again, yet I have no trace of emetophobia at this point in time. Aversion to foods that have made you sick in the past is an "old" human characteristic from an evolutionary perspective, so much so that it has become instinctive. Even the great apes will avoid any plants or leaves that they ate before *the thing* happened, in case they've eaten something that was poisonous. My patients are always relieved when I tell them that setting a goal to eat something that made you sick is not a "relevant" goal. Note that this is not the same as having a goal to eat foods that have never made you ill. If you're simply afraid that you could get food poisoning from potato salad, but have never tried it, then trying potato salad would be a good example of an attainable goal.

You may wish to set a goal for yourself to stop taking anti-depressants or anti-anxiety medication. Some people want to set goals never to begin. But are these goals actually relevant? It is possible that part of your phobia is a chemical issue in the brain, in which case medication may be the only treatment that will make a significant difference to your anxiety level, and you may never be able to fully recover without it.

Several patients I've worked with have wished to go through pregnancy without any medication for morning sickness or, for that matter, any pain medication in labor such as an epidural. I like to remind them that it's the 21st century—people don't need to suffer in pregnancy or in labor or at all when there are perfectly safe and effective medications to treat pain, nausea, and chronic anxiety.

Explore your goals to check if they're relevant and write your answers in Figure 1.5.

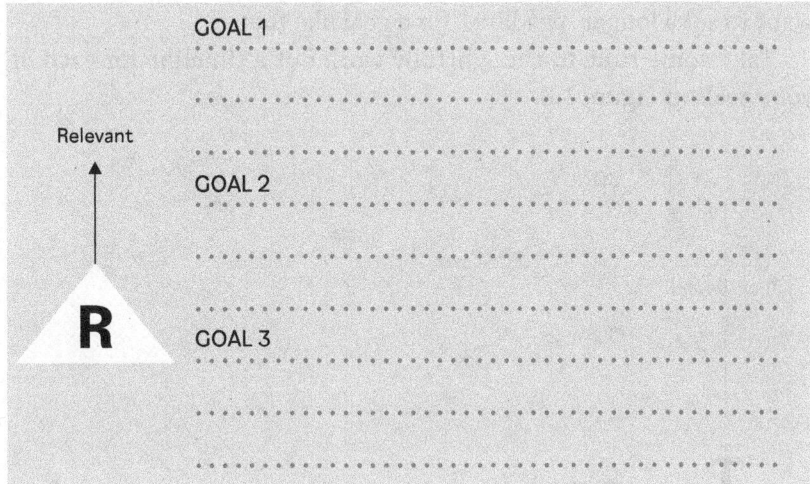

Figure 1.5. Relevant

Time-bound

How long does it take to overcome emetophobia? I'm always surprised when a family member, such as a parent of a child I'm working with, comments that they're not getting any better after they've been working with me for only a couple of sessions. There is no quick fix to most of life's problems, not least of which is a serious, debilitating condition like emetophobia.

Sometimes people in my Facebook group announce that they need to do something frightening for the first time, such as go to a party or fly somewhere on vacation. Then they ask the group if we have any "tips or tricks" to help them. I know it's an expression at this writing, but I want to throw my laptop at the wall every time I hear the words "tips and tricks." There are none. Nada. Not one trick. There is only a long, deeply involved process that includes dedication, commitment, and hard work. So let's be realistic about the amount of time we need to achieve our goals. I like the term of two years. That's the amount of time it took me to start eating normally again the '70s, and it was also the amount of time that it took me to fully recover from emetophobia in the 2000s. If you can break down your goals according to the SMART formula, you may be able to set some very specific and realistic timelines to achieve them. How long will it take you to be able to eat at a restaurant? Perhaps a month or two. Perhaps you think you could do it tonight. Perhaps you can't even imagine it, in which case you'll want to set a longer "deadline" for a goal like that.

Take some time to thoughtfully work out a timeline for each of your goals in Figure 1.6.

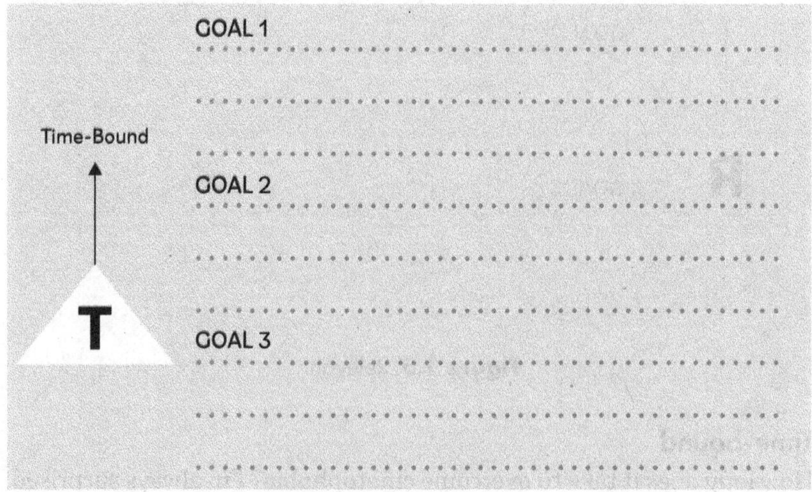

Figure 1.6. Time-bound

Now let's begin recovery!

THE LADDER

Think of emetophobia as if you've fallen down a deep, dark hole. Your life may feel that way right now. But there is light at the top and from this light you can see a ladder going all the way up (see Figure 1.7). Each rung of the ladder represents one small, easy exposure exercise. The top rung of the ladder, finally taking you out to the world above, the world you're currently missing out on, would be something such as feeling very ill yourself or being around someone who is ill. You may think you can never climb this ladder, but that's because you're at the bottom of the hole right now. You may be wandering around, unaware there even is a ladder.

Don't skip to the end of this book, look at the last few exercises and think *I could never do that.* Think about how impossible it would be to reach the top rung of the ladder from where you are now, at the bottom of the hole. Even halfway up the ladder it's impossible to get to the top rung without going up each rung separately. Yet, when you're standing on a rung, any rung, you are safe. You can easily keep climbing; you just have to hold on and go up one rung at a time. So never mind what's at the end of this book, as that's like the top of the ladder. Concentrate instead on that first rung.

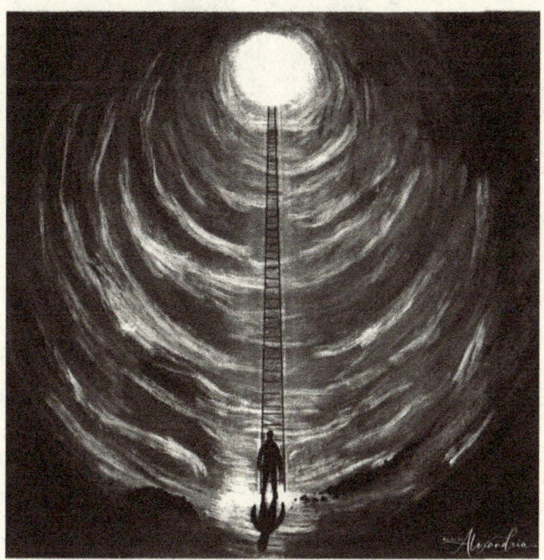

Figure 1.7. Person in a hole with a ladder

Source © E. Alexandria Bois 2025

Measuring anxiety

Before we start climbing, we need a way of measuring our progress. This is normally done in CBT with a scale we call the SUD scale, which stands for "subjective units of distress." (Some therapists use the word "discomfort" instead of distress.) I use a scale that goes from 0–10, where 0 represents no anxiety at all and 10 is the *worst panic possible*. Since 10 is as bad as it can possibly get, there is no use reporting 11 or 3000 or any other number higher than 10.

The most important word in SUD is "subjective." This means that the number is yours and yours alone. Someone who reports a 6 might be sweating, crying, and wringing their hands, whereas someone else would not experience those symptoms until 8 or 9. Nevertheless, most people report their numbers close to what is indicated in Figure 1.8.

Being able to identify what SUD number you're experiencing at any given time is critical to your recovery.

Subjective units of distress
10 Panic attack
Dissociation
9 Crying, pacing
8 Hard to tolerate
7 Very distressed
6 Urge to run
5 Heart racing
4 Very worried
3 Fidgety
2 Nervous
1 Unsettled
0 Calm, happy

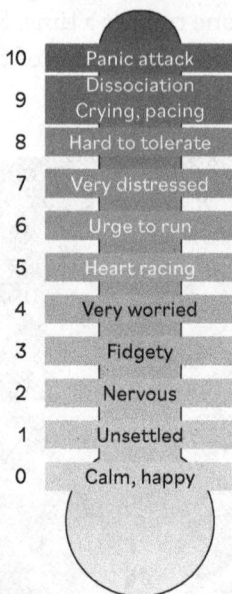

Figure 1.8. Sample SUD scale

Nausea levels

If you have trouble with feeling nauseous, especially if nausea triggers you, then try recording your nausea level from 0–10 where 0 is feeling perfectly well and 10 is actually doing *the thing*. Each time you do an exposure exercise, record your SUD number from 0–10 as well, where 0 is perfectly calm and 10 is the worst panic possible.

TIME TO START CLIMBING

The first rung of the ladder is to see *that word*. I understand that the word may make you very uncomfortable. Perhaps you conjure up an image or a memory when you see the word. Perhaps you're afraid it will be "burned in your brain" and you will think about it for the rest of the day, or you won't be able to sleep tonight. You may believe that seeing that word, much less staring at it for several minutes, will somehow "jinx" you and you will become ill yourself. Allow me to let you in on a little secret: *there is no such thing as a jinx.* Sure, there are coincidences. Someone reading these first few pages may indeed be ill later. But that would be a coincidence, not a jinx. Jinxes can be traced back to 17th-century folklore about spells and sorcery. I'm going to take a guess that you don't believe in spells or sorcery. Some of you may even follow religions that outlaw all such beliefs. So why pick this one ancient thing to believe in and have it affect everything you do, including tossing aside a book that may help you? Trust me on this—there is no such thing as a jinx, or Santa Claus, or the tooth fairy.

Looking at the word may make you slightly anxious, but it won't be too bad. You will be able to tolerate the small amount of anxiety that arises from seeing it spelled out. You may think that you cannot, but you can. And when you do, you will be so proud of yourself because it will open a whole realm of possibilities for you—from reading social media posts and books, to listening to podcasts, to talking with a therapist about your emetophobia and working toward your recovery. Besides, aren't you anxious a lot of the time anyway? How much can one little word really matter?

Let's grip that ladder and start climbing so you can read the rest of this book. I promise you that it is possible. After all, you're just staring at a word on a page. Nothing will happen to you except that you will feel either a tiny jolt like a static electricity shock or you will feel slightly uncomfortable. The word may "trigger" your discomfort but feeling it will not hurt you. We don't like feeling discomfort, but unfortunately, we must experience it in life from time to time, and recovering from the phobia is one of those times. Eventually, you will be able to experience more and more, but those are rungs near the top of the ladder, so you don't need to worry about them right now.

EXERCISE 1: Working in imagination

Begin by writing down your SUD number between 0 and 10 as to how much anxiety you feel right now. This number is called a *baseline*. Remember that 0 is no anxiety and 10 is the *worst panic possible*.

Do not try to control your anxiety during this or any of the exercises in this book. That means no purposeful slow breathing, no relaxing, reassuring yourself with your inner thoughts, and definitely no safety behaviors like sipping water, eating mints, etc. You want to feel the anxiety and leave it alone, letting it come down on its own.

Now think about the word. Just the word. Think of its five letters. Spell them in your head. Envision it. Take a moment to do that.

Now think of what the word means. In English it can be either a noun or a verb. Think of it as a noun, what it looks like. This can be very uncomfortable, but you can do it.

Now think of the word as a verb, an action. Who is doing the action in your mind? Is it you or someone else? Try to picture it, along with the word.

Think about what happened in your body during this exercise. Did you notice how it felt when your anxiety became higher? Note down any body symptoms you may have had, such as elevated heart rate, sweating, tight chest or legs, and so on.

MEMORIES

Exercise 1 (imagining the word) may have raised a memory for you. This is very normal, but you may have been trying to avoid such memories for a long time because they made you uncomfortable or scared. You might have been thinking that the memory would make you do *the thing*, but that is wholly impossible. It is the avoidance of your memory, the fighting against remembering it, that makes you anxious, not the memory itself. If every time you have the memory you reach for a safety behavior like medication or water or gum, then all you are doing is keeping the memory frozen in that scary place.

Allow me to tell you something about our memory system and to illustrate it with a story. Our brains do not remember facts; they only remember feelings, and we fill in what we believe are the facts as we recall the memory. Most people don't realize that this is a scientific thing, and so two life partners may fight about the real version of events.

Brad Gushue won the first Olympic gold medal for Canada in men's curling in 2006. My memory of watching it on TV is crystal clear. He called his mother on the phone back in St John's. When she finally answered, he said, "Mum? I just won an Olympic gold medal," and he broke down in tears before he could even finish the sentence. I've told this story *exactly* this way many times since then because I remember it so clearly. About a month ago (now 20 years later), I saw there was a YouTube video of this phone call. To my shock and surprise, I hadn't remembered it very well at all. He called his home and asked his brother to "Put mum on." When she answered, he said, "Well, we did it." Then he listened for a bit, thanked her, and told her, "I've gotta go because I'm about to be interviewed by the CBC." The reporter asked him what it was like to talk to his mother at home, and *that* was when he burst into tears. He made a comment like, "I don't wanna be a sook [suck]," and laughed. The only things in my memory that were correct were the emotions involved: a proud phone call to his mother, the crying. The rest I just filled in, and quite incorrectly!

What does this mean for your memories that are being triggered by things you imagine, even if they're just words? It means that what you remember probably didn't even happen that way. The only thing valid is that you were scared. The rest you very well could be making up right now. So you don't need to be afraid of remembering that memory. Remembering it won't hurt you in the least. All it will do is raise your anxiety a bit, which we call "being triggered." But if you don't do anything to try to lower the anxiety or calm down, if you just sit there, then it will go away on its own and you will no longer be triggered by this memory. But you have to do *absolutely nothing*. No slow breathing, no trying to relax, no reassuring yourself, no using your senses to ground yourself, and absolutely no safety behaviors like walking around, sipping water, or hugging your dog.

OLD-SCHOOL ANXIETY TREATMENT VS. NOW

Were you able to tolerate that anxious, uncomfortable feeling? Your previous therapist or other books you've read may contradict the idea of allowing your anxiety to rise without trying to control it or lower it. If so, they are not familiar with the latest research on anxiety treatment, especially exposure therapy. Some therapists are afraid to do any kind of exposure with their patients, or they are afraid of letting them experience anxiety and doing nothing about it. I used to be one of those therapists myself. Research on anxiety in the past decade or so, particularly in what we call "second-generation CBT," has shown us the benefit of allowing your anxiety to be with you for a time. Your brain needs to learn that you're not in any danger by thinking about *the thing*, and it will only learn that you are in no danger if you do nothing and think nothing. It's like the part of your brain that is sending you "danger" signals says to itself: *She's not doing anything. She's just sitting there, so I guess this isn't a dangerous situation after all.*

Acceptance and Commitment Therapy (ACT) is an example of an evidence-based, second-generation CBT and it is quite popular with therapists today. Research has demonstrated that trying to calm down when you're anxious may help you in the moment and it may help you for a while, but it won't ultimately help you overcome an anxiety disorder, including emetophobia, once and for all because you'll have to continue doing it or the fear will return. Second-generation CBT therapies, such as ACT, work on the principles of something known as *inhibitory learning*, which has been scientifically studied at length. Ready to try it?

EXERCISE 2: Exposure—Seeing the word

Record your baseline SUD level.

Look at the first picture on the website by using the QR code below. Record your SUD level (higher or lower).

If lower, try the Raise Game (Chapter Two). If higher, ask yourself if you can tolerate the discomfort of the anxiety without avoiding the picture, reaching for a safety behavior or reassuring yourself.

Keep looking at the picture and tolerating the discomfort until your anxiety naturally goes down to the baseline or lower.

After imagining the word and allowing your anxiety to calm down by itself, you should be able to see the word behind this QR code.

http://emetophobiahelp.org/figure-1-9

Now it's time for us to print the word here so you can see it in the book (on the next page).

VOMIT

Did you feel a little rush of adrenaline like a jolt of electricity when you saw it? That's okay—it won't hurt you. Go back and look at it again, and think about what it means, both as a noun and a verb. Allow your anxiety to rise a bit. It won't go too high. It should peak in a few moments and then start to fall on its own.

EXERCISE 3: Exposure—Interacting with the word
Write the word "VOMIT" in large letters with a thick marker pen on a piece of copy paper. Make a few duplicates. Tape them up around your house, especially in your kitchen and beside the washroom mirror. Put one in the hallway. Every time you pass it, say the word out loud and think about what it is. Ask family members to do the same, if you're within earshot.

Ask family members to use the word "vomit" as many times as they can, even in silly ways, for one week. The dinner table is fair game.

Write the word out 50 times in your own handwriting (typing it won't help).

Write 10 sentences using the word.

When seeing, hearing, and saying the word become so mundane that you're literally bored with it, you can take the papers down, congratulate yourself, and treat yourself to something nice like some time alone with your dog or a purring cat. If you don't have pets, perhaps go sit somewhere you can enjoy nature for a short time.

LET'S KEEP CLIMBING

Back from your nature walk or from cuddling your pet? Great! It's time to go up one more rung of the ladder. Although I will only use the word "vomit" in this book, there are many other words that mean the same thing, and you will usually hear other words more often than the word "vomit" as it is often only used in medical settings. Your parents probably taught you something else when you were young. The terms they used will either trigger you (raise your anxiety slightly) worse than the word "vomit" or they will be easier to see. Everyone is different in that regard. These words and phrases may be very difficult to look at, but try to do it without any safety behaviors. The words or phrases get slightly harder as you go along, but don't skip over any. Take careful note or write down both your baseline anxiety number from the SUD and any number higher for each of the slides of words found by scanning the QR code below.

EXERCISE 4: Exposure—Interacting with other words

Do the same with all these words as you did with Exercises 2 and 3.

Record your baseline SUD level.

Look at the first picture on the website by using the QR code below. Record your SUD level (higher or lower).

If lower, try the Raise Game (Chapter Two). If higher, ask yourself if you can tolerate the discomfort of the anxiety without avoiding the picture, reaching for a safety behavior or reassuring yourself.

Keep looking at the picture and tolerating the discomfort until your anxiety naturally goes down to the baseline or lower.

http://emetophobiahelp.org/figure-1-10

SUMMARY

- You set goals for yourself that were Specific, Measurable, Attainable, Relevant and Time-bound (SMART).
- I described emetophobia metaphorically, as someone who has fallen down a hole, but there is a ladder up to safety.

- Exposure work is like going up the ladder one rung at a time.
- You need to measure your anxiety level with a SUD (subjective units of distress) scale from 0–10, where 10 is the worst panic possible.
- When feeling anxious, try to leave the anxiety alone and don't seek to lower it in any way, even by reassuring yourself. Wait for it to come down on its own.
- The first rung of the ladder to climb is to see the word "vomit" spelled out.
- First you worked with the word in imagination, then you looked at it behind a QR code, and then you looked at it written in the book.
- I demonstrated how our memories are not reliable.
- You interacted with the word "vomit" as an exercise. You then looked at and interacted with other words that also mean "vomit."
- You rewarded yourself with a comforting time alone.

Chapter Two

EXPOSURE AND RESPONSE PREVENTION

For most people with emetophobia, even the word "exposure" conjures up their worst nightmare. Many believe that if you have to do exposure to overcome the phobia, then they would rather keep the phobia. In all my years of listening to and speaking to people with emetophobia online on social media, in person, or over Zoom, I have come to believe that those who want to avoid exposure therapy usually don't know what it is or how it should work.

Some therapists have contributed to the misunderstanding of exposure therapy because they misunderstand it themselves. In misunderstanding it, both they and their patients have the idea that exposure means you have to vomit. This is not true. Not only is it not true, but researchers and therapists who *do* understand exposure therapy now know that vomiting not only doesn't help but it can bring harm and even retraumatize the patient. So we never, *ever* recommend vomiting as a form of exposure.

Significant others and family members may be partly to blame as well. They might be quick to say, "You just need to vomit once and you'll be fine." You won't be fine. Well, you'll be fine physically, but emotionally you won't be. On the other hand, those who have gone through ERP therapy may elect to make themselves vomit if they wish. Or they can wait 12 years, like I did, for it to happen naturally.

ERP is about starting with your foot on the first rung of the ladder and going up very slowly, making sure that you've got your footing before you continue to the next rung. The second half of this sentence may be the most important: *you have to feel safe and secure on the rung you're on before you continue to go up.*

Dr. David Russ and I have an ERP ladder on our free website for therapist resources.[1] Every once in a while a patient stumbles upon the site and decides to race up the ladder, clutching their phone with one hand and the arm of a chair with the other, knuckles white, barely breathing. "I'm fine with all those words and pictures," they'll tell me. "I'm fine with" is not the point, though. Almost anyone with a fear of clowns can freak out every Hallowe'en when they see one, run the other way, heart pounding, and next Hallowe'en they'll be just as frightened of the clowns, and if they don't pay attention they'll soon stop going out on Hallowe'en, going to parades, or watching anything on their phone or TV in case they see a clown.

You've already put your foot on the first rung when you finally looked at the word "vomit" and then did all the exercises in Chapter One. Wait...did you do them? Or are you saying, "I'm fine with looking at words. All I'm afraid of is feeling nauseous and vomiting?" You have totally missed the point.

What I'm most interested in is whether that anxiety number moved up the SUD scale from your baseline. Before you looked at the words, did you write down a baseline number of how much anxiety you were feeling already? Then, when you looked at the words, did the number move at all? The exercise works if the number goes up a little. And soon I'll explain what to do if it doesn't go up.

Why are all these numbers so important? You can probably handle a lot of those numbers already. Probably from 1–5 is where you are almost every day. To explain, I'll need to take a little detour here so I can show you in the simplest terms possible how the brain works and, more specifically, what is happening in the brain of a person with emetophobia.

YOUR BRAIN MADE EASY

Made easy? The human brain is the most complicated thing in all of the known universe. Scientists have mapped a lot of the brain, but not all of it, and still cannot explain to us simply if our minds, our

1 www.emetophobia.net

consciousness, and our brain activity are all the same thing. Nevertheless, allow me to try to show you what's happening in your brain right now.

Not that long ago, brain scientists explained that the brain had three essential parts: the brainstem, the midbrain, and the neocortex. So if you adhere to the theory of evolution, the brainstem is the oldest part of our brains (often called the "reptilian brain"), the midbrain we share with other mammals, as among other things it regulates emotions, and the neocortex (neo means "new") is the newest part of our brains and that which is unique to humans (Figure 2.1).

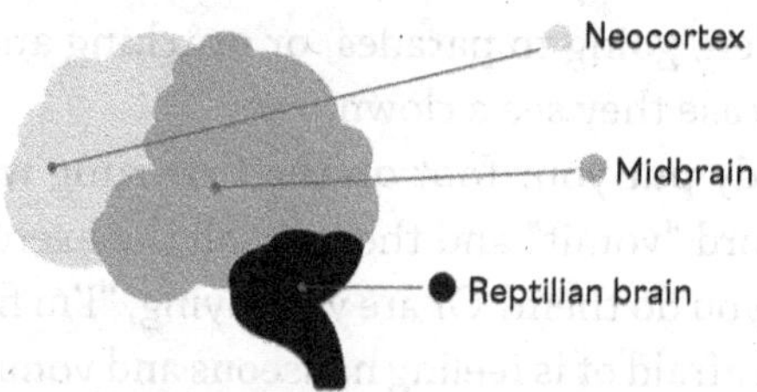

Figure 2.1. The three-part brain

In reality the brain has many parts, almost like little organs all squished together over time. All the parts are connected by "wiring" known as neuropathways, where electrical signals jump from cell to cell. These neuropathways are a little like computers except that brains also have things like blood, oxygen, hormones, and other chemicals running through them. All the parts of the brain are connected into sets of various systems. So the brain isn't really triune—it actually has many systems. There isn't just one part for memory, for example. Various parts are included in the system for memory.

But for our purposes, let's look at these three parts and focus on two of them in particular. The midbrain, near the brainstem, contains two little organs known as the amygdala. You may have heard or read about the amygdala and its function in the fear system. The amygdala is responsible for your survival, so it's super-important. It is also connected intricately to the memory system, so if we remove it, you'll be in a *Groundhog Day* movie for the rest of your life. Instead of amygdala, and since they are near the brainstem or reptilian brain, let's make it memorable by calling it the *lizard brain* from now on (see Figure 2.2).

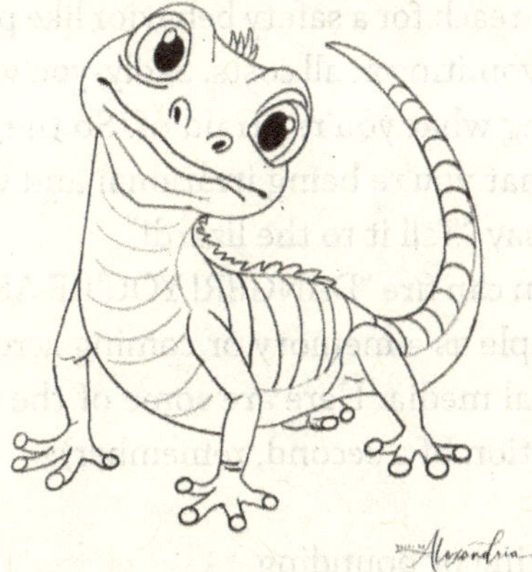

Figure 2.2. A lizard
Source © E. Alexandria Bois 2025

The lizard brain has but one message that it signals to you: "DANGER! YOU'RE ABOUT TO DIE ANY SECOND!" The lizard brain doesn't know much else. Could you teach a lizard to do tricks? Yes, if you withheld its food and rewarded it with food, and didn't get too close to it when you were holding its food, and if you trained it for a long, long, *long* time.

For some reason (and so far we don't know why) your lizard brain is sending you the "DANGER!" signal whenever it gets triggered by something to do with vomit. That may be stories, pictures, videos, or any number of grumbly feelings in your tummy. The problem is made worse by the fact that the lizard brain fires that signal to your body in just a fraction of a second. I once read that it fires in 1/5000th of a second. It may not be quite that fast, but it's definitely faster than having a thought.

The *neocortex* at the front of your brain is responsible for things like logic, reasoning, organization, mathematics, and so on. Have you ever had someone try to give you a logical argument as to why you should not be afraid of vomiting? Have you ever tried to give *yourself* this logical argument and wondered why it didn't work? The answer is simple. You *already know* that vomiting isn't dangerous and it's part of our human experience and nobody dies from it. In fact, it's meant to make you feel better: to rid your body of deadly poisons and toxic viruses. But knowing these facts isn't enough because your lizard brain doesn't "know." It's already very worked up long before you even realize, logically, what is happening. It has prepared your body for fight-or-flight.

You run away. You reach for a safety behavior like peppermint or ginger so that you avoid vomiting at all costs. Sadly, you've now reinforced the phobia by avoiding what you're afraid of. So the next time someone tries to tell you that you're being irrational and vomiting won't hurt you anyway, just say "Tell it to the lizard!"

The lizard brain can fire "DANGER! YOU'RE ABOUT TO DIE!" with something as simple as a memory or coming across a word in a book or a story on social media. Here are some of the ways your body can respond (in a fraction of a second, remember):

- Heart—racing or pounding
- Breathing—short, shallow, or holding the breath
- Tightness, discomfort in the chest or chest pain
- Tight muscles (shoulders, jaw, legs)
- Butterflies in the "stomach" (adrenalin)
- Adrenalin rush ("stomach drops," "whoomf" feeling, or a jolt, like electricity)
- Dizziness or light-headedness
- Nausea (queasy, churning or tight or painful stomach)
- Clenching the jaw or teeth
- Jittery—tapping of feet or anxious fingers or twitching
- Shaking
- Hot flashes or heating up; cold sweats or chills
- Weakness, lethargy or fatigue
- Pacing back and forth or restlessness
- Reaching for a safety behavior, such as medication or water or gum
- Running away or putting fingers in ears
- Anxious chatter or going silent
- Anxious nail biting, hair pulling, or skin picking
- Urge to self-harm (cutting, bruising)
- Crying or fainting
- Intense focus or obsessive, repetitive thoughts
- Loose stools or diarrhea
- Headache and/or blurred vision
- Dissociation from reality or tunnel vision
- Feeling of impending doom or horror
- Racing thoughts ("What if..."/OMG).

Once you experience any of these body responses, as a person with emetophobia, you're going to get even more anxious because you believe that they don't only indicate you're about to die but also that you're about to vomit (even though that isn't true).

The most common symptom people with emetophobia misinterpret is nausea. Once your lizard brain signals danger, one of the things it does is to stop the digestion process. This is because digestion takes energy, and you need that energy to run away from the danger. There isn't any danger, though, because vomiting isn't dangerous, but your lizard brain doesn't know that. It triggers your fight-or-flight just the same way it would if you encountered a grizzly bear in the woods or a serial killer running after you with an axe.

BACK TO ERP

ERP is really the only way out of emetophobia because you need that lizard brain to be triggered, but not too much, in order to begin teaching it that there is nothing to be afraid of. You can undergo cognitive therapy alone (trying to change your thoughts) or "talk therapy," but without the lizard brain being activated and thus involved you will probably not get very far, or if you do, it won't last. Exposure therapy, done properly, will expose you little by little to triggering things so that your lizard brain is activated and becomes part of the exercise. If not, that lizard is just sunning itself on a rock, asleep. If the exposure exercises are too difficult, then your lizard brain will be screaming "DANGER" so loud you can't hear anything else. It has the ability to slow down or completely shut down your neocortex altogether, which is bad news because you need to be able to talk and think logically.

Gradual exposure or variability?

Gradual exposure means just that, gradual. Slow. Easy. Exposure exercises should begin just as we have in this book, with the word "vomit," and progress to other words that mean the same thing. Then progress to sentences and paragraphs, and then perhaps stories. Patients should write the stories themselves.

Current research on ERP shows that developing a hierarchy (or a ladder) with exercises going from easiest to most difficult is not as effective as variability, which means mixing up easy and hard exposures.

The problem with that is I could not imagine getting a person with emetophobia to agree to it. Can you imagine if your therapist said, "First, I'll show you a word, then maybe a picture of someone projectile vomiting, then a drawing, and who knows what's next?" You'd probably politely decline or run screaming from the room. I know I would. I would never have agreed to some sort of "surprise" exposure exercise. In fact, I reassure my patients that I would never, ever, do this.

This is not to say that the concept of variability (from the same root as "variety") in exposure therapy is unimportant. In order to achieve variability, I have my patients go through a gradual hierarchy of exposure exercises and then, if they feel ready to do so, they can look up pictures and videos of vomiting on the internet to get the benefit of this latest research. Try not to think about that now. It will be much easier when you finally get to that exercise.

IS VOMITING REALLY HARMLESS?

You may have heard of someone who died from vomiting, but I promise you, they were unconscious at the time and lying on their back. They were either passed out from drink or drugs, or they were somehow actually unconscious. You cannot die from vomiting if you're conscious. I seriously doubt that any person with emetophobia is going to get passed-out drunk, as most of you will be too afraid to drink at all because you've all seen that drunk people vomit all the time.

You can't choke on vomit either. Choking, real choking, means that your airway is completely blocked such as with a piece of food; this you can die from, although it's rare. But you cannot choke on vomit because there is a little flap that covers your airway when you vomit. Some vomit can get into your airway as it opens, but this will make you cough, so you cough it up. We've all had a little water or food or even saliva "go down the wrong pipe" and had a fit of coughing. This has nothing to do with choking, dying, or vomiting. Little kids might vomit from a coughing fit, but their throat and windpipe aren't fully formed yet. Adults will not vomit from coughing—especially those of us who really don't want to.

Every once in a while we hear about someone who aspirates vomit into their lungs, and it causes pneumonia, which can be a dangerous condition. These people are either very young or very old or very sick.

The average healthy adult does not need to worry about aspiration pneumonia at all, so put it right out of your mind.

You may feel as if you can't breathe if you vomit. You may remember this sensation, but I assure you that you can certainly breathe. Vomiting takes 2–3 seconds. Anyone can hold their breath for 2–3 seconds. But I understand why you may feel this way. Remember that little flap I just told you about that closes when you vomit? Well, it closes over your airway. While it is doing that, in those 2–3 seconds, many (anxious) people feel that they cannot breathe, which is true, but you don't want to breathe in those 2–3 seconds when vomiting is happening anyway. It can be a scary sensation, momentarily, but I promise you that within 3 seconds you can take a deep breath, even if you vomit again a few seconds after that.

You can't die.

You can't choke.

You can't suffocate.

That lizard brain of yours is grossly misinformed about vomiting being dangerous. I tell my patients all the time that vomiting is *normal*, *natural* and *neutral*. Normal, because everyone does it (including most mammals). Natural, because it's part of nature that's there to save your life or help your body feel better. Neutral because it's neither 100 percent good nor 100 percent bad. It's not all good because nobody likes it. Nobody hopes they wake up one day and spend that day vomiting. Most people truly hate it. It's gross, it feels awful, your stomach really hurts beforehand, and it leaves you with a terrible taste in your mouth. But it's not *all* bad because a lot of people prefer to vomit than to feel nauseous all day. It's not all bad because it saves you from poisons and toxins and millions of viral particles replicating in your stomach after you contract a virus.

MY FIRST ERP THERAPY

My hunt for a professional who could help me began in 1981 when I finally told my doctor that I was "terrified of sick people and sickness" (I still didn't have the guts to say it was only vomiting). He was very kind and referred me to a psychiatrist who I'll just call Dr. B. As he was very kind and this was the '80s, I figured I could be straight with him, praying that he didn't have me committed. Dr. B. talked with me, tried imaginal stuff (which didn't help), and administered the Minnesota Multiphasic Personality Inventory (MMPI), a standard personality inventory that apparently would have shown if I needed to be committed. He raved about my results, as if I had aced a history test. "You may have a phobia, but you have such a good personality," he beamed. By "personality" he wasn't referring to what you or I would mean by the word. He meant psychopathology. I was unimpressed by whatever he was impressed by, and it took me several decades to realize that this "impressive" personality type I have is what led me to overcome emetophobia virtually by myself. Not everyone has a personality type like this, but it doesn't matter anymore. It is now up to us, as a psychotherapist community, to offer solutions to people with emetophobia despite a wide range of personality types, strengths, and weaknesses.

After two years of not being able to help me, Dr. B. became aware of a study being conducted in a Vancouver hospital by a psychologist named Dr. H. Clare Philips. There would be 10 sessions of exposure therapy conducted in a group setting. The group was all people with emetophobia, although not even the researchers used that word at the time. Everyone there was afraid of vomiting. I was eight months pregnant.

The program began with an evaluation. I was told to stand at the end of a long hallway leading to a washroom that had vomit on the floor and asked to walk as far as I could toward it. I clarified with the researcher that there were no people in the washroom. No problem. I walked right in. For the next test I was told that they were going to start a video of someone vomiting, they'd start a stopwatch, and I could say "stop" at any time. I told them not to even put it on—that I couldn't watch any of it—which is why I was there. They told me they had to start it but I could say "stop" at any time. As soon as an image came into view I screamed "Stop!" and burst into tears. I shook and sobbed uncontrollably. You have to remember that in 1983 there were almost no movies and no TV shows with vomiting in them, no internet, no YouTube. I had literally not seen anyone vomit in years and didn't know what would happen if I did.

Before treatment began we were given three cassette tapes of relaxation through guided imagery, also called Progressive Muscle Relaxation (PMR). Each was about 20 minutes long and we were to listen to them once a day. Being a keener, and off work at the time,

I listened to them three times a day. The idea, we were told, was that you couldn't be relaxed and panicked at the same time. I thought this was odd because I knew that I could be relaxed one second and panicked a hundredth of a second later. But I complied because I have one of those personalities, I guess. The treatment consisted of Dr. Philips showing us a video, in black and white, where she was seated in a chair with a garbage can beside her. She looked nauseous. I remember that we watched more and more of the video each week and had to fill out a form with how much anxiety we felt, 0–10, and how much nausea, also 0–10. Eventually, the video showed Dr. Philips putting her head in the garbage can and making vomit noises. The next video showed her interviewing a man who put his head into a garbage can at one point and "vomited." We saw the video clips several times.

I don't remember what my scores were each time, but I clearly saw that my nausea score and my anxiety score went up and down together. I remembered Mother's voice in my head whenever I said I felt sick (a pain here, an ache there, a gurgling, indigestion, gas, being full, being hungry): "That's just your digestive system working as it should," she would say, or "That's probably gas." I put two and two together and somehow, remarkably, I began to be less and less afraid of vomiting myself. By the end of the group exposures, it was as if a lightbulb had come on and I came to assume that I would probably not vomit 99 percent of the time when I thought I might. By the time 1985 rolled around I was happily pregnant again with my third child.

In 2020, when I began to study research articles on emetophobia I came across Philips' (1985) published study.[2] When describing the assessment she wrote, "one patient had a panic attack after [watching the video for] only .05 seconds!" That was yours truly, Anna S. Christie. *You were the worst of the worst* I said to myself when I read it. Ironic, don't you think?

LOSING MY FEAR OF VOMITING MYSELF

After taking part in the exposure group with Dr. Philips, I slowly stopped fearing being sick myself. It was probably always there,

2 Philips, H. C. (1985) "Return of fear in the treatment of a fear of vomiting." *Behavior Research and Therapy* 23, 1, 45–52. https://doi.org/10.1016/0005-7967(85)90141-X

somewhere in the background, but it didn't emerge unless I was truly about to vomit, which would turn out to be very, very rarely.

I have tried to recreate how getting over this fear happened for me in order to help other people with emetophobia, most of whom fear themselves vomiting more than they fear seeing others, but I can't put my finger on how it worked for me. Perhaps it was just the last link in a long chain of events that led me to believe that I wouldn't be sick most of the time anyway. Perhaps it was memorizing all the little urps and burps and pains and rumbles that Mother had an explanation for in my digestive system. Don't get me wrong, I'm still sure that fearing being sick myself underlay all my emetophobia fears and it went as far back as my brother's and later my father's death, both of whom were "sick" before they died. But I could function in the world and as a mom. I had a career and a family, friends, hobbies, and a social life. As long as the kids weren't sick, I was perfectly fine. But little by little, the fear of seeing them, or anyone else, be sick seemed to grow and grow until it had ballooned into a giant problem.

THE TEST FOR MYSELF, 13 YEARS LATER

It's hard to know whether you're truly over your fear of vomiting yourself until it actually happens. It wasn't until 1996 for me, when my two youngest kids were just 13 and 11, on a Saturday evening in October when I felt the lump in my breast. It was a hard lump, and I was shocked at the size, given that I did breast exams every month and it hadn't been there the month before. I'd also been having mammograms for five years, since my sister had breast cancer.

Tests quickly confirmed that the lump was malignant, and I was looking at some of the most feared experiences of a person with emetophobia: surgery *and* chemotherapy. Surgery was the first hurdle. I think my mind had gone back to the old days of putting people under general anesthetic with ether—they were all sick upon being woken up. Or perhaps I remembered my sister after her surgery five years earlier. But all those times I had said to myself *I'd rather die than vomit* had come now to a place where the rubber hit the road. It didn't take me more than an instant to look into the faces of my children to realize that I did not want to die at 37 and leave them without a mother. I would fight with everything I had because in that moment, looking death right in the face was infinitely more frightening than vomiting. You probably think you're different than me, and that you really and truly would rather die, but brain science tells a different story.

The day of surgery arrived. It was perfectly timed to the exact day my husband was writing the bar exam. Imagine that for a moment. As I was waiting to be wheeled into the operating room the anesthesiologist came to see me. She was a pleasant, grandmotherly woman who reassured me that she would be with me the whole time, watching over me. I told her I was terrified of vomiting when I woke up, so she reassured me that she would give me anti-emetic drugs while still asleep, and order more for when I awakened. The first thing I said when I was awake was "I feel sick." I'm not sure I did, but it says a lot about how much of my emetophobia was left, despite Dr. Philips's group therapy 13 years earlier.

The nurse in the recovery room gave me Gravol® (Dramamine®) in my IV and I felt instantly better. The rest of my recovery was a piece of cake, but the biggest obstacle still loomed ahead: chemotherapy. It had made my sister terribly sick, but she also didn't feel her family was able to pay the $30/pill for the then-experimental drug Ondansetron (Zofran), so she suffered through the vomiting.

When I got to the chemo room with my husband, I was shaking, tearful, and seriously reconsidering the whole thing. The worst part was walking in and seeing a row of chairs with other people in them receiving chemo. I burst into tears, turning to my husband and the nurse saying, "I can't do it! I can't be here with all these other people!" I didn't know at the time that people don't actually vomit while they're receiving chemo—it takes a few hours after you get home to affect your stomach lining and trigger the vomiting switch in your brain. The nurse quickly replied that she could move one of the chemo chairs into a small closet-like room that was used for previewing videos by the staff. It had a TV and one of those VCRs that played the brick-sized VHS tapes. For the next three treatments, I brought my set of *Fawlty Towers* videos to watch.

After my first treatment, they sent me home with two or three different kinds of anti-emetics that had weird side-effects, like shaky legs syndrome and bed sores after just a few hours. None of them helped the nausea and I was miserable and scared for about three days until my stomach lining grew back. I didn't vomit. Someone (you know about *those* people) told me that each chemo treatment gets progressively worse, so I was terrified for the next three weeks until I saw my oncologist again and completely broke down. He told me that he could prescribe Ondansetron, but that drug plans didn't cover it and it was $30/pill. I said I would sell my car if I had to (I didn't). He also told me that I could take Gravol® in between the dosages of Ondansetron. Coupled with taking my chemo in that closet, I managed to get through all four chemo treatments with no vomiting and little resulting anxiety. The best was yet to come.

Once a few days had passed after my fourth and final chemo treatment I thought I was home-free. But I developed an infection, which is pretty common with chemo patients. My doctor prescribed an antibiotic that I had taken a few years before with no problems or side effects. But only a few minutes after I took the first pill I felt nausea like nothing I can ever remember experiencing before and an incredible pain in my stomach. I paced back and forth at home, fretting and freaking out for about an hour. Finally, I resigned myself to the inevitability of it, went to the washroom and vomited. Immediately, the thought in my head was, *Well that was a big fat nothing.* My next thought was, *I can't believe I wasted so many years of my life being scared of that.*

My chemotherapy was over, and while radiation treatments exhausted me beyond belief, they didn't cause any nausea. From that day on, I never thought about vomiting myself at all. But unfortunately, the trauma of cancer made my fear of seeing, hearing, or being around anyone else who was vomiting rise to a ridiculous level. Every bump in the night from my kids, every person who looked pale, any talk of a virus going around and I went right back to being a sniveling lump of jelly. Learning to breathe and relax when my anxiety went up through Dr. Philips's group had worked, but the effect had not lasted. I still had work to do, and I had no idea how to go about finding out how to do it. We still had no internet at home.

NEW RESEARCH

Some therapists are still using PMR with their patients with phobias, including emetophobia, although few patients find it ultimately helpful in the long run. A newer methodology for treating anxiety is called Acceptance and Commitment Therapy (ACT), which is referred to as "second-generation CBT." ACT is about tolerating or *accepting* the anxiety when it arises, and just being uncomfortable but not trying to fix it. So you don't try to breathe, relax, or reassure yourself with any sort of logic that you won't be sick. You just leave the anxiety alone and allow it to be there. I ask my patients to give me a SUD number when their anxiety goes up, and then I ask, "Can you tolerate that number without trying to change or lower it?" Very rarely does anyone say "no."

The other important piece of ACT is that it's important to *commit* to living your life according to your values, even if you're anxious or afraid. Having an understanding, first, of what you value in life is important to get clear on, so let's now try an exercise.

EXERCISE 1: Establishing your core values

Look at this sample list (in alphabetical order) of core values, and circle those you consider to be your top five:

- Charity
- Earth
- Faith
- Family
- Freedom
- Friendship
- Fun
- Generosity
- Health
- Honesty
- Integrity
- Justice
- Kindness
- Learning
- Legacy
- Money
- Precision
- Responsibility
- Safety
- Success
- Work

When you are deciding what to do instead of a safety behavior when you are anxious, try to carry on living your life according to your values. This can be as simple as doing the dishes or spending time watching TV with your partner because you value things like family and responsibility before anything else. If you value things like money, success, and work, you will want to work instead of pacing the floor or lying in bed with a hot water bottle.

Now, I want to say here that if anyone had told me to approach my fear of vomiting this way at the start, I would have left their office and never come back. That's because I believed at the time that I could *not* tolerate the anxiety because it seemed to come upon me instantly and go from 0 to 10 in a millisecond. Which it did. I haven't really met anyone like me, exactly, in this regard. One colleague suggested that perhaps I have poor emotion regulation, and at first I balked at that idea because I don't get angry and fly off the handle or cry at the drop of a hat, but when I think back on my life, I certainly used to. I would get instantly angry at times, and I couldn't even argue a point in a meeting without tearing up. But I've had over 300 hours of psychotherapy not related to emetophobia now, so I handle life as a much more mature and wiser person. (I figured this was important work before becoming anyone's therapist.)

So as a person with essentially poor emotion regulation, I can testify that when your anxiety skyrockets to 10 out of 10 on the SUD scale, this is something we call a panic attack. During a panic attack, your neocortex (thinking brain) slows down incredibly or shuts down entirely. You can't even think about what you're supposed to do when you panic. Fight-or-flight is now fully engaged, in an instant, and you will seek to avoid the situation by running for the hills, or you will anxiously grab a safety behavior like an anti-emetic, gum, mints, ginger, or all four. You may pace back and forth crying and screaming at everyone around you to help, even though they can't possibly.

This first-hand knowledge of panic attacks has led me to conclude that few people can "tolerate" anxiety at high SUD levels. I have found in my clinical practice that some people can tolerate 8 out of 10, but most people can only tolerate 7 while staying in the frightening situation. The numbers 9 and 10 are out of the question for most people. So at these high numbers, the technique has to change to one of breathing slowly, especially on the exhale, and relaxing all the large muscles in your body from head to toe. Once you bring your anxiety down to a tolerable level you can cease the relaxation and breathing exercises and just accept the uncomfortable feelings that go with anxiety below 9.

Progressive Muscle Relaxation (PMR)

To use PMR to help you calm an intolerable panic attack down to a level you can tolerate you have to practice it when you're *not* anxious. When I say practice, I mean like an Olympic athlete or a professional pianist. Listen to a guided imagery recording, such as the ones in Exercise 2, once a day for about three months, or twice a day for six weeks. Remember to listen when you're already fairly calm. They won't help you to calm down if you're anxious—you're going to do that yourself once your body knows how to do it automatically, and I've found that this takes at least 90 repetitions of the exercise. Some people may be able to master it in less, particularly if they're used to meditating. Others may not learn the skill after 90 times, and may have to listen several hundred times.

EXERCISE 2: Listening to PMR recordings

This QR code will take you to my YouTube channel for relaxation recordings. If you don't like the sound of my voice, or if you get bored with these two recordings, there are hundreds more on YouTube. Just be sure to listen to one that uses guided imagery, going from head to toe, as opposed to relaxation recordings with just the sound of rain or waves.

https://www.youtube.com/playlist?list=PLbpiDcZKaOTSs10vwSCzFgeh_W0oWowLj

MY STAR PLAN

My STAR plan integrates the principles of ACT (tolerating or accepting the anxiety) with the principle of PMR when your anxiety reaches intolerable levels. Don't feel bad if it does. Your therapist may consciously or subconsciously shame you for not being able to tolerate it, saying such things as "It's *just* anxiety" or "You have to face your fears." I am very careful now with my patients in saying anything like "It's just anxiety" because I remember the judgmental sound of that word "just." The thing is, emetophobia is one of the trickiest phobias to treat because deep down, or maybe not very deep down, a person with emetophobia believes that if they get anxious enough they will vomit. This is because they've seen anxious (or "nervous") people on TV vomit before they go on stage and such. But people with emetophobia don't vomit when they're anxious. Just like everyone else, they get nauseous because their digestion slows down or stops, but they simply put up with it. People without emetophobia who feel like that go in the washroom and vomit and then say they feel better (which makes sense—nothing is in their stomach now). But someone with emetophobia would not even entertain the idea of vomiting to feel better. We will put up with a boatload of nausea before we would ever do that. I promise you, if you have emetophobia you will *not* vomit when you're anxious. As your SUD level goes up, your feeling of impending vomit is stronger and stronger, so you think if you "tolerate" that feeling and don't do anything about it that you'll be sick for sure. But you won't. I'd bet money on it, because there's no risk involved in that bet just as there's no risk involved in you vomiting from anxiety. You, as a person with emetophobia, must be literally poisoned or overwhelmed with viral load and very sick in order to vomit. We'll get to that later. Meanwhile, here's my STAR plan (Figure 2.3).

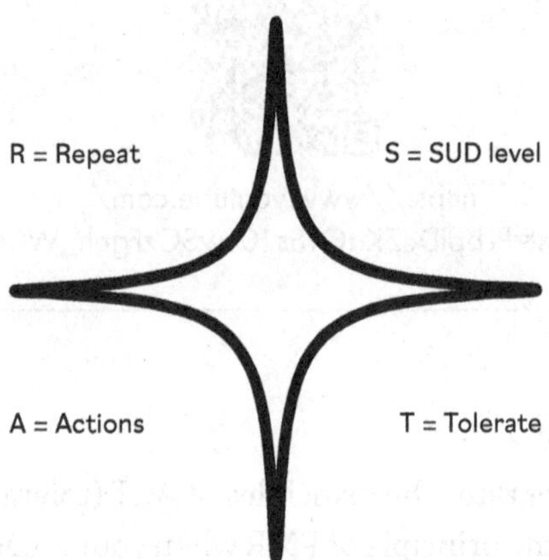

Figure 2.3. My STAR plan
© Anna Christie 2022

The "S" stands for "SUD scale" or "subjective units of distress," as explained in Chapter One. The first and most important question that you must ask yourself when becoming aware of being anxious is "What number am I at on the SUD scale?" This helps you to determine what to do.

The next question you must ask yourself is the "T," which stands for "tolerate"—can you tolerate this number *without doing anything* to try to change it or lower it? Your therapists in the past may have told you to breathe and relax when you feel anxious, but modern research has shown us that this will mean you have to keep doing it for the rest of your days. Normally if the number is 7 or below it is tolerable for most people, but don't beat yourself up if you can't tolerate 7. What does "tolerate" even mean? It means you can live with the amount of discomfort that this amount of anxiety causes in your body. You don't have to like it, but you can accept it. You can also ask yourself at this point "Can I accept any outcome from having my anxiety at this level?" What if the outcome is vomiting? You will probably know that anxiety at 7 or below does not result in vomiting, even if you're afraid that it might if it goes higher. It's still a good question to keep asking yourself. At first, the answer will probably be "no," but you will slowly and surely move toward a "yes" response to that question of accepting any outcome.

If you *cannot* tolerate the SUD number, then the next question to ask yourself is "What actions can I take to calm down?" "A" stands for "actions" in the STAR plan. Actions must begin with slow, slow breathing and not holding your breath at either the top of the inhale or the bottom of the exhale. Just keep it going. Slowly, slowly. Be especially mindful of the exhale being as slow as possible. Some schools of thought teach a different way of breathing that might include holding your breath at one point. I don't recommend that, because when you hold your breath, your heart rate automatically goes up.

The QR code below leads to a little video showing my heart rate being quite high and the effect on the heart rate of just one or two slow breaths and of keeping your air moving.

https://youtube.com/shorts/p4GFKkQUu_I

THE RAISE GAME

Some of you reading this book will have already done exposure work with your therapist or on your own. You may have read other emetophobia self-help books or seen our resource website for therapists and its exposure pictures and such. You may be bored with the exercises so far. So just for you, here's something else you can try. I call it the "Raise

Game" because I have a sense of humor and it's not a game after all because it's not even fun; it's just an emetophobia exercise.

In the Raise Game, you begin one of the exercises such as looking at words or writing sentences or a story and you *purposely make your anxiety go up.* This "game" becomes really important later on when your lizard brain will try to make up a story about a drawing or picture so that it becomes less scary. But becoming *less* scary is not the idea. You need to get a little bit scared for exposure to work properly. If you tell yourself, *That's just a drawing, so it can't hurt me or make me sick,* then your lizard brain won't activate at all. It won't learn anything because it's not even present in the class. Your lizard brain has to show up, which means it has to send you at least a little bit of a "DANGER!" signal. Only when you remain in the scary situation (still looking at the picture) and *do nothing* (tolerate or accept the anxiety level) can that ol' reptile learn anything, and all it needs to learn is that there is no danger in the situation, meaning that vomiting is not dangerous at all and so you don't need to be afraid of it.

THE DAWN OF THE INTERNET

Around the turn of the century we finally got a dial-up connection for our computer so that we could access the internet. It was a wild and untapped realm of reality. There was still no YouTube, or even Google images. Images were not indexed in any easy way that one could find them. There was also no social media, so communities had not yet begun to form in this new, untamed land.

Search engines were in their infancy, so Google was just beginning to break free of the pack. Once it did, I came to thinking one day that since there were a number of people in the group with Dr. Philips who had the same phobia, perhaps I could find some information about it that my searching in libraries had failed to produce in the past. So I simply typed the words "fear of vomiting" into this new Google thing. You could count on one hand the number of hits that came up, but one stuck out immediately: the International Emetophobia Society (at www.emetophobia.org). It was (and still is) an online discussion forum. Although their popularity has waned since Facebook groups became a thing in the past decade, I discovered two things that day that would aid my healing immensely: my phobia had a name, and I had found others like me.

It was through this group that I began to put together items of gradual exposure to help with both my recovery and what I would eventually compile to help others. It all began with a woman named Margaret from the Netherlands who was computer-savvy and she designed a little website with pictures. Each picture was behind a "door" with a title and a description on it that had to be clicked to get to the picture. They started with just a funny picture of some eggs with faces drawn on that were cracked in the middle and the yolk was spilling out, which faintly resembled vomiting. I could look at a few of them myself, but others I had to have my husband print out and put them in an envelope for me to take to my therapist.

By the mid-2000s, as I found more and more pictures and information on the internet, I was able to set up a rudimentary website of my own on a little Weebly site. I set up two separate sites with a link on the first to the second (emetophobiahelp.org and emetophobiaresource.org). The resource site had the first hierarchy on the internet for people with emetophobia to use with their therapists. There were words, sentences, paragraphs, and a few pictures along with a list of movies with vomiting scenes that you could rent at the time on VHS tape. My own healing journey continued by watching these movie scenes up to 100 times—I'm thinking specifically of the blueberry pie-eating contest in the movie *Stand By Me*. One hundred times. I finally stopped reacting to it, even by the tiniest bit, which was my goal.

THE NEXT RUNG ON YOUR LADDER

EXERCISE 3: Exposure—Reading sentences

You are now ready to try reading some sentences with words in them that mean the same thing as "vomit." You'll find these sentences by using the following QR code. Start by jotting down your baseline anxiety number from 0–10, where 0 is no anxiety and 10 is the worst panic possible. If you wish, write down how much nausea you feel as well, 0–10.

Read each sentence out loud and think about what it means. Picture the scene. Now notice the number your anxiety has gone to (if it has moved). Can you tolerate this number? Can you accept any outcome? If your anxiety does not go up at all during this exercise, try the Raise Game.

https://emetophobiahelp.org/figure-2-6-sentences/

EXERCISE 4: Looking at cartoons

Once you have been able to read the sentences without your anxiety going up (even if you try by using the Raise Game) you can use the QR code below to look at cartoons of silly situations or drawings of cartoon characters that look unwell.

https://emetophobiahelp.org/figure-2-7-drawings-nauseous-characters/

SUMMARY

- Many people with emetophobia fear exposure therapy, believing it requires them to vomit, but this is a misunderstanding. Proper Exposure and Response Prevention (ERP) is a gradual process that never involves vomiting, and instead helps retrain the brain to reduce fear responses.
- The amygdala, or "lizard brain," is responsible for detecting danger, and it misinterprets vomiting as a life-threatening event, triggering intense fear and physical symptoms.
- Vomiting is unpleasant but not dangerous. Common fears of

choking, suffocating, or dying from vomiting are based on misconceptions. The body has built-in protections that ensure vomiting is safe. It takes less than 3 seconds of your life.

- ERP is the most effective treatment for emetophobia because it engages the lizard brain and teaches it that vomiting is not dangerous. Gradual exposure, done in a slow, controlled way, is the only evidence-based therapy proven to work for emetophobia.
- I participated in a 1983 research study that used ERP to treat emetophobia. Exposure to videos of simulated vomiting helped lower my fear of nausea and being sick myself, while my fear of seeing others vomit got better initially, but then much worse over time.
- A cancer diagnosis 13 years later showed me I really would rather vomit than die, although I never did vomit through surgery or chemo.
- When I ultimately experienced vomiting, I realized it was "a big fat nothing."
- The internet connected me with others with emetophobia, including one person who developed structured exposure tools, such as images and videos.
- A key technique in ERP is intentionally raising anxiety slightly during exposure exercises to ensure the brain learns. If anxiety doesn't increase, the exercise is ineffective.
- Modern research supports Acceptance and Commitment Therapy (ACT), which encourages accepting the discomfort of anxiety rather than trying to control or lower it. ACT also teaches that we need to commit to living our lives according to our values.
- My STAR plan offers a structured approach to managing anxiety. The goal is to tolerate and accept anxiety rather than eliminate it.
- The chapter concludes with beginner exposure exercises, such as reading sentences with vomit-related words and looking at cartoons.

Chapter Three

SAFETY BEHAVIORS

A safety behavior is any action you take to stop yourself from vomiting. It can be as simple as reaching for a sip of water, or as subconscious as reassuring yourself you won't be sick. To get over emetophobia completely you will have to give up every single one of your safety behaviors in order to convince that lizard brain that you don't need anything to keep you safe because you are safe, even if you vomit.

Avoidance is a safety behavior in and of itself. You might have a long list of people, places, and things that you avoid, and often there are items on your list that would surprise the people around you. Everything you avoid is for the purpose of keeping yourself "safe" from vomiting.

I have an interesting history with safety behaviors. Perhaps being born, growing up, and raising kids before the internet was a gift to me. I imagine if I'd found some of the Facebook groups that are out there now, with other people with emetophobia, my life might have taken a different trajectory. As a young child, Mother would "help me" to diagnose my various stomach twinges and such, and, being the queen of self-medication, she would offer me some sort of remedy. If it was gas, she'd give me Tums® or Pepto-Bismol® or Gravol®. I think it was easier for me to give up my safety behavior of over-the-counter (OTC) medicine because every single time I vomited, I had taken one of them beforehand. So it became infinitely clear to me that they didn't work. There were no prescription anti-emetics that I was aware of in those days either. Also, for some reason, I never believed that I was sick when I wasn't sick. Mother had taught me well that gas is just gas, cramps are just cramps, heartburn is just heartburn, overeating is just overeating. None of it led to vomiting. And again, my nausea when I became anxious was fixed when I was in that exposure group and saw the nausea numbers (not just for me—for everyone else as well) go down when the anxiety numbers went down.

No one ever told me about ginger or mint, and nobody in the '60s "sipped" water. We drank water out of the tap or from a water fountain, one glass at a time. We also knew nothing about noroviruses—what caused them or how they were transmitted. We washed our hands when they were dirty. Like digging-in-the-garden dirty. My kids had norovirus a couple of times that I remember. My husband looked after them and neither of us ever caught it from them. Ignorance is bliss in the case of emetophobia. My other safety behavior was one that many anxious people have: bargaining with God. (I explain more about it in point #16.)

Since some family members and friends of people with emetophobia will read this book, I will list safety behaviors here and try my best to explain the reasoning behind each of them. Place a checkmark beside each of the safety behaviors you use. If you see something you haven't previously thought of, *don't* start doing it! You're trying to get over your emetophobia, not make it worse.

SAFETY BEHAVIORS

1. Mint

People with emetophobia use mint in various forms to keep themselves from feeling sick: essential oil, mint candy, mint gum, and mint tea, to name a few. Some sniff peppermint oil when anxious (nauseous). Some people with emetophobia have sucked on so many mint candies that their teeth are rotting, and they're generally afraid of the dentist because they're worried about gagging. In reality, no amount of mint will stop someone from vomiting. It is a mild help for an upset tummy or a bit of gas. Most mints don't even contain any actual mint.

2. Ginger

Ginger comes in the form of candies, tea, raw ginger (to make tea or add to other edible items), soda pops (the strongest ginger concentration of which is found in ginger beer), as well as pill form. Gravol® has a "non-drowsy" pill that is just concentrated organic ginger. I don't know how effective this is compared to the regular drug containing dimenhydrinate, or whether there is a strong placebo effect in taking it. Ginger can also exacerbate acid reflux and/or cause heartburn. At one point the most popular ginger ale maker (Canada Dry) was criticized because there was no ginger in it. Since then they've changed the formula to contain some amount of actual ginger, although some people allege that it's not even enough for a human to taste.

3. Sipping water

I'm not sure how people with emetophobia got the idea that sipping water helps with nausea, but it's probably somewhere on the internet. Many people argue with me that they shouldn't stop because water is good for you. To an extent, yes, water is good for you, although an excess of water can also be harmful and can even cause nausea and vomiting. I often recommend that if people with emetophobia are using this as a safety behavior in order to stay hydrated, that they drink an eight-ounce glass of water every two hours instead of carrying around a water bottle with them like a security blanket.

4. OTC medications

There are so many OTC medications for an upset stomach it makes you wonder what on earth is wrong with our digestive systems in the Western world. There are medications for gas, bloating, overeating, acid reflux, heartburn, nausea, constipation, flatulence, diarrhea, and just about everything in between. The more often you take these OTC meds, the less effective they become.

5. Prescription anti-emetics

People with emetophobia generally believe that Ondansetron (Zofran) is the be-all and end-all in anti-vomiting drugs, probably because it's given to people who are undergoing chemotherapy. I think that the picture of people undergoing chemo being miraculously cured of their vomiting with just one drug is what makes up the myth of Ondansetron. Resisting the temptation to get too technical here, allow me to just say that different anti-emetic drugs work on different parts of the brain's nausea and vomiting systems. Some work on a particular part that is sensitive to chemicals (chemotherapy). Others work on the inner ear (motion sickness), some with morning sickness (hormones), and still others work for problems right in the stomach (viruses). There is another part of the brain involved in nausea and vomiting, however, and that is the front of your brain where you're sensing and thinking about things, especially disgusting things.

Some emotion systems in the brain trigger vomiting in some people. Overeating or drinking too much (such as those fools who tried to drink a gallon of milk when the stomach only holds about half a gallon) can also trigger the body to vomit. This is why there are so many different types of anti-emetics on the market and doctors (pharmacists and anesthesiologists in particular) are very familiar with all of them and how they work. So, long story short, your Ondansetron does not work to prevent vomiting in every single situation. Doctors who prescribe it to people with emetophobia are not doing them any favors. It helps with chemo, it helps with post-surgical nausea (even though there are many other, better drugs), but it isn't the first go-to drug for motion sickness or morning sickness, and it only has a placebo effect for nausea caused by anxiety.

6. Checking your temperature

Constantly checking your temperature, as a healthy adult, is a wholly unnecessary behavior. By the time you contract a fever you'll have many other symptoms of illness anyway, and fevers are indicative of lots of things besides norovirus. It's often helpful to check the temperature of a child or an elderly person to see if they might have a serious infection that they can't tell us about, but otherwise there's no need to even keep a thermometer in your house. If you have kids and want to keep one around for them, though, give it to your partner to hide for you rather than throwing it out.

7. Asking for reassurance

This can take many forms, from asking "Do you think I'll be sick?" to "Does this chicken look cooked to you?" to "How do *you* feel?" It is always a safety behavior. Asking needling questions of your significant other or children falls into the same category. I've had many a patient who asks their children how they feel on a daily basis. This kind of anxiety may not lead your children to have emetophobia necessarily, but it may lead them to have some sort of anxiety problem.

8. Throwing out food

Most people with emetophobia throw out far too much food. They often won't eat something even before the "best before" date printed on it, or they won't eat leftovers at all. It's rare for someone to get sick from food prepared in small quantities at home. Eating a bite of spoiled food seldom, if ever, results in illness.

9. Overcooking food

Please don't serve your poor family dry, rubber chicken (or pork, fish, or anything else). Get yourself a good digital thermometer and download a chart on how to cook food to the proper temperature.

10. Googling

When you have emetophobia (or illness anxiety), Google is your worst enemy. You always think that you can Google something to reassure yourself and make yourself feel better, but it never works that way. You know I'm right, don't you? People with emetophobia Google all sorts of things, from norovirus outbreaks to symptoms of diseases that could make you vomit. Even if the norovirus outbreak isn't in your neighborhood, just seeing that it's anywhere (and it's always somewhere) is anxiety-producing. It doesn't matter where the outbreaks are or aren't.

People with emetophobia also spend an inordinate amount of time Googling symptoms they feel they have, wondering if they'll lead to vomiting. Google won't help you with that, either, as I'm sure you know by now if you're doing it. Let me save you some time: *every drug* will list nausea and vomiting as a potential side effect. Yet people with emetophobia don't vomit often or easily. We would have to be poisoned or overloaded with viral particles to get sick. You need not even concern yourself with any other reason you may find by Googling.

11. Behaviors and rituals

As emetophobia is related to OCD, many of us can have odd behaviors and/or rituals that we believe will keep us from vomiting. Some people swallow, spit, burp, bite their cheek, and all manner of other overt or subtle behaviors. Others have rituals that they believe will keep them "safe" from vomiting, such as touching wood, sitting or lying down a certain way, switching lights on and off, etc., etc. Of course these are all just habits or superstitions that do not prevent vomiting or anything else "bad" from happening.

12. Excessive cleaning and handwashing

Upon this writing in early February, a patient just sent me a picture of her hands that were red and raw from washing them. Despite always having safety behaviors and cleaning rituals, she contracted norovirus last fall anyway. This could be because hands that are rough and raw are more likely to trap norovirus particles in them that won't wash away, so you need to only wash your hands at the following times: after using the washroom, when coming in from outside, before eating (particularly with your hands), and before preparing food. That should be a maximum of 10 times in a day. Any more than that and you're sipping too much water and using the washroom too many times.

People with emetophobia also tend to do a massively unnecessary amount of cleaning of their homes, offices, and cars. If everyone in your home washes their hands when they come in from outside, there's no need to habitually clean everything with harsh chemicals. If someone in your home is sick, confine them to one washroom only. After they recover and for the following two weeks be sure to wipe flusher handles, faucets, doorknobs, countertops, and light switches with a bleach solution.[1]

Some people wipe down airplane armrests and tables, and reclean their entire hotel room. This is completely unnecessary. Just don't put your hands in your mouth and enjoy your vacation.

13. BRAT diet or restricting food

BRAT stands for "bananas, rice, applesauce, and toast." It's a very bland diet that is suggested for folks who have either just overcome an illness, or who have had surgery and are transitioning from clear fluids to full fluids to BRAT before adding in other foods. Many people with emetophobia have taken this BRAT diet and run with it, restricting their food intake to only those foods, or even less. This is especially true if they think they've been exposed to norovirus, which is often. Having had norovirus a couple of times in my life I can assure you that

1 One teaspoon of bleach to one quart or litre of water is the recommended mixture to kill viruses. If you use a tablespoon of bleach to one litre/quart of water you are using three times too much bleach.

vomiting something is a lot better than vomiting nothing. Restricting oneself to bland foods such as bananas, rice, applesauce, and toast is what you do *after* you've been vomiting and you're transitioning from clear fluids to solid food again. It doesn't help you in the least if you've ingested enough viral particles to be sick.

14. Grape juice and/or apple cider vinegar

Neither of these prevent or kill norovirus. This is 100 percent a myth. You should not give grape juice to your children in the hope that they won't catch the virus. Children shouldn't be drinking juice at all, as it's full of (natural) sugars and suppresses their appetite for solid food, which has many more nutrients. Kids should be drinking water 99 percent of the time so that when you take them out that one special night for a root beer float, their eyes light up like the sun.

15. Mental (internal) reassurance

People with emetophobia often seem resistant to CBT because the therapist is unaware that they're using their internal voice as a safety behavior, and as long as they do that they can't get fully over the phobia. Your internal dialogue may sound something like this:

> You're okay. It won't make you sick. You felt like this last Tuesday, and you weren't sick. Just breathe. Try to relax and breathe. It's been 48 hours already since you were exposed. But you have good hygiene so it's unlikely you caught anything from them and besides, you didn't even go inside the house. If the kids get sick you can go to your mother's.

I may not have covered it all in that last paragraph, but you get the idea. Self-reassurance, self-soothing, self-coaching, even self-hypnosis—these are all done, ultimately, not only so that you calm down but also so that you won't vomit.

Every time you catch yourself saying soothing things to yourself, tell yourself to stop. I used to say, "Stop it Anna!" Sometimes the same thought came back an hour later, at which time I would tell myself to stop again. Eventually I got tired of yelling at myself inside my head and these thoughts stopped coming. This technique does not work for everyone. In Chapter Six I will talk more about what to do with the annoying thoughts that keep coming to you again and again.

16. Bargaining

My father was a minister, and so I have gone to church almost every Sunday of my life. For 30 years, I was the minister. As a theologian, I know that God isn't all that concerned with little problems like harmless vomiting. God has bigger fish to fry, like the plight of the poor, the marginalized, the dying, wars, famine, climate change, and so forth. Nevertheless, as a person with emetophobia, I bargained with God continually, especially as a child. My knees were blistered from the time I spent on them, praying. I know now that God had no intention of entering into my bargains. I promised to be good, to love my neighbor, to obey the commandments, to be nicer to Mother, and eventually, to get help for my phobia. I can't even remember the amount of bargaining chips I offered up to God if only I were offered the protection of not vomiting and never being near anyone else who did. The problem with such prayers (and all prayers that beg God for anything) is that they don't always work. Once I was in theological college I came to believe that these were the futile prattle of human beings, and God wasn't interested in any of it. I am still a Christian, and I still pray and believe in its power, not to heal us from human disease as individuals, but rather its power to heal all of humanity.

My point is that you may be literally *using* God for your own ends if you're praying not to vomit. I once read about a man with emetophobia who was an atheist, but still he bargained with the universe itself.

17. People watching

Normally when people with emetophobia are in a crowd, they scan it looking for people who may be unwell. I remember spending a great deal of time doing this when I was a kid and even as a young adult. It didn't matter if it was at the mall, at a kids' birthday party, at a concert or a movie or even in a meeting. I was looking for pale people, sweating people, or anyone holding their stomach. You probably have a keen sense for knowing what to look for as you've likely had a lot of practice.

EXERCISE 1: Scanning for sick people

Turn this habit around by sitting on one of those benches in a shopping mall and watching people go by, noticing only their shoes. Think about how expensive or cheap the shoes might be, how pretty they are or are not, and whether you think the shoes match the outfit the person is wearing. Don't look at anyone's face. Just the shoes, and maybe their clothing. Journal about how this exercise made you feel. Now go back and try it again, looking for signs of sickness in people. Journal about how you feel after spending the same amount of time watching people as when you were looking at their shoes.

I'm quite sure you already know that the second exercise will make you feel more anxious. However, even if you know that, you must still *experience it*, or your lizard brain won't learn anything. Knowing intellectually that it's better to watch people's shoes than look at them for signs of sickness will not help you in your recovery. Do the exercise! Do it several times. Then make up your mind that whenever you're in a crowd of people you're going to look at their shoes unless you need to interact with them face-to-face. Even then, notice their hair, their facial features, their clothing—anything but whether or not they look sick.

WHAT IS A SAFETY BEHAVIOR VS. COMMON SENSE?

I get asked this question in every single class I teach, or some variation of it, such as, "What if it's just good hygiene?" These questions make perfect sense, and sometimes it's hard to tell the difference. Sometimes, you will have a friend or family member who is clean and neat, washing their hands after washroom use and before cooking, but that person would not be considered a germophobe. My son-in-law was trained as a high school biology teacher, so he knows how to keep a clean and sanitary kitchen and so on. The difference is that all his behavior is based solely on facts and not on anxiety. If you wash your hands because it's just a normal thing to do, and you're not anxious, that's fine. But if you are anxiously washing your hands, then it may be a good idea to "swing the pendulum in the opposite direction so it comes to rest in the middle."

The swinging pendulum metaphor means that you should try *not* washing your hands before you eat with your hands, for a whole day, perhaps. Sometimes, people without emetophobia (let's call them "normal" for a moment) have to do this and they don't give it a second thought. Sometimes I need to eat a sandwich and I'm not near a sink, so I just eat it and think to myself, *Oh well, usually the worst doesn't happen.* Trying this on for size reminds me of a saying I coined: *If you want to be normal you have to act normal.* Find some "normal" people and shadow them for a day. Wash hands when they do. Eat what they eat. You will probably find this very difficult to do at first.

GIVING UP SAFETY BEHAVIORS

The patients I work with and the people who take my classes have many safety behaviors, apart from all the things they avoid.

EXERCISE 2: Safety behaviors calendar

You can do this exercise simultaneously with all the exposure exercises under QR codes in this book, or you can do all the exposures and then circle back to this exercise for safety behaviors. Note: you can do this exercise with a spreadsheet, sorted by your numbers 1–100, in order of easiest to most difficult, and an online calendar if you wish.

Make a list of all your safety behaviors (avoidance behaviors will be discussed at length in Chapter Seven).

Give each behavior a number between 1 and 100, without using any number more than once—1 represents the easiest thing to give up or stop avoiding and 100 represents the most difficult.

Put your list in order from 1–100 (easiest to most difficult).

Print out three blank monthly calendars and write in all the dates.

Put each of your behaviors on one day of the calendar. It's up to you how you do this, and it may depend on how many safety behaviors you have. You may only have 12 and you're willing to give up one every week. You may have 24 and you're willing to give up two each week, or you believe you can give up 10 of them right away and then distribute the other 14 over the three months.

A perfect hierarchy isn't necessary. As I have said, researchers have concluded that doing harder exposures and then easier ones might be more effective. I don't recommend this with pictures and videos, but you can try it with your safety and avoidance behaviors if you like.

Chapter Four will discuss support persons. If you have one at this time, it's important that you share your calendar with them so they can check in with you and hold you accountable to completing them.

EXERCISE 3: Exposure—Pictures of nauseous people

Now it's time to do some exposures that look at real people as opposed to cartoons or drawings. But don't worry, this exercise is just looking at pictures of people who feel nauseous or people *before* they vomit.

Record your baseline SUD level.

Look at the first picture on the website by using the QR code below. Record your SUD level (higher or lower).

If lower, try the Raise Game (Chapter Two). If higher, ask yourself if you can tolerate the discomfort of the anxiety without avoiding the picture, reaching for a safety behavior or reassuring yourself.

Keep looking at the picture and tolerating the discomfort until your anxiety naturally goes down to the baseline or lower.

https://emetophobiahelp.org/figure-3-1-people-before-vomiting/

SUMMARY

- I listed the most common safety behaviors and discussed why they don't work.
- If you want to be normal, you have to act normal.

- I showed that internal self-reassurance is a safety behavior.
- I talked about my own safety behaviors of stomach meds, avoidance, and bargaining.
- You made a list of your avoidance and safety behaviors, put them in order, into a hierarchy, and created a three-month calendar for giving them up.
- You looked at pictures of nauseous people and tolerated the anxiety until it went down on its own.

Chapter Four

GARNERING SUPPORT

Your best chance at beating emetophobia using only a self-help book like this one is if you have a good support network. While a whole network is best, just having one support person in the house with you will go a long way to helping you. Ask them to begin by reading this book themselves, or work through it with them, chapter by chapter.

FAMILY

When I was growing up as a kid with emetophobia I had no support whatsoever because I couldn't bring myself to tell Mother what was wrong with me or what I feared. I found out years later that she knew I was terrified of vomiting and sick people, but because the phobia was so severe she assumed that I had to have something else going on as well that I just wouldn't admit to her. She was honestly mystified. My only sister, who was 21 and married when dad died, assumed I was just a spoiled brat who wanted attention. She was angered by her belief that Mother just let me get away with everything because Mother used to beat her with a strap as a kid for the smallest of indiscretions.

I don't know why I couldn't talk to Mother about my true fears. I think I was terrified that someone would make me "face my fears" somehow, maybe by putting me in a room with someone vomiting, or giving me ipecac to drink, perhaps secretly, so I'd vomit so badly I would die. I had heard that expression "You have to face your fears" many, many times growing up. The thought of it at the time made me literally numb with fear. To me, my whole problem was that I *couldn't* face my fears. The fear was just too strong. If I was in any situation whatsoever that involved vomiting I was having a full-blown panic attack. Ten out of ten anxiety, which is the worst panic possible. The feeling would come over me in a millisecond. It started with a huge whoosh of adrenaline that sent my heart instantly pounding and I was overcome with a feeling of doom—like I had been captured and tied up by a known serial killer and my murder at any moment was completely inevitable. The whole scene was like a mass murder to me, with bodies and blood everywhere. It was horrific and terrifying all at the same time.

What I have just described is what I think "You have to face your fears" meant to me every time I heard it. Needless to say, I don't use this expression with my patients—ever! It's not wrong or untrue; it just carries a lot of baggage with me, and I don't want to impart that kind of thing on anyone else. The first half of the phrase "You have to" is as bad as the second. It's like someone is giving me an order, forcing me into something against my will. *I'll show you—I DON'T have to* was what I thought. *I will run—far and fast. Hide if I must. And if you find me and drag me back there I will fight you to the death.*

Once I met and married my husband, and he knew about my phobia, things got to be a little easier, although he really had no idea how to support me fully and neither did I. I was grateful that he looked after the kids when they were sick, so long as they got sick when he was home. Most of the time if I called him at work to say one of the kids was sick he would come home from work (an hour away), but he was never very happy about it. He did expect me to clean up vomit, wash sheets in the middle of the night, and bring the child a glass of water in the washroom if he called for it.

He put up with the fact that our bedroom door had to be closed and locked at all times so I could sleep. I was always scared that a child would come in to tell us they didn't feel well and would vomit inside the room while I was asleep. So they knocked on the door and my husband jumped up to look after them. If they made it to the washroom, in later years, I would lock the door again, get back into bed and plug my ears until I couldn't help but hear him knocking loudly on our door to get back in. So he did supportive things, but with great frustration.

I remember when we went to Disneyland I wouldn't go on any rides with him and the kids. At one point he said to me "Anna, you're just no fun," and it made me the saddest I had ever been as a parent. I knew I wasn't a "terrible mother" as many of my patients despair about, because the kids were always well taken care of by him if they were ill, and the rest of the time by me. I was very focused on my career, but I loved the kids more than life itself, and still do.

Shame is also a big part of the reason I could never tell anyone about my phobia. I recall one time, shortly after dad died, I was sitting on Mother's knee, so I would have been nine or ten. I wanted to tell her about my phobia. The words "I'm afraid of people vomiting" were right on the tip of my tongue, but I could not spit them out. A lot of my patients and the people with emetophobia I talk to online feel the same sense of shame. Sometimes, this comes from people belittling the phobia by saying that much-despised, "Well, nobody likes it." I'm not sure what that means, exactly, when people say it to someone with emetophobia. Do they mean that you're just like everyone else and don't have a phobia at all? As if they would know this and you wouldn't. Or maybe they mean that no one likes it, but other people aren't acting crazy like you are about it. Whatever they mean, it's one of the most unsupportive things people can say. I remember a nurse in the hospital Emergency Room (ER) one time writing notes on my chart. I said I had a phobia of vomiting and all she did was look at me, furrowing her brow in a quizzical way, and I died with shame. She didn't believe it was a real phobia and didn't have any sympathy for me whatsoever. Again, very unsupportive.

In a few ways, I was blessed by the fact that I couldn't bring myself to tell anyone about my emetophobia until adulthood. Blessed, only in that Mother couldn't enable any of my fears as she did by accommodating my school refusal. When dad died we moved to his old hometown of Kincardine, Ontario. Mother found an apartment over a drug store downtown. School was a very short walk down the street and around a corner, about two city blocks. She must have walked me to school on the first day, which was in February of Grade Five. After that, I would get very anxious and insist that she walk with me every day. Sometimes she would get to the corner where the post office was and I would say it was okay that she went in and checked for her mail rather than continuing up the next street with me. I don't know why some days she could walk me to the post office and other days she had to walk me all the way to school—perhaps I didn't feel well on the more difficult days. I do know that one day I insisted that she walk right into the school with me and hand me over to the teacher when I was in Grade Six. She was upset about that, and I could feel her anger. That never happened again.

Part way through Grade Six Mother got the job of school secretary, so the situation with walking me to school promptly ended. My anxiety was very much lessened once Mother was present at school all day, although I never needed to go into the office to see her. Over the next two-and-a-half years to the end of Grade Eight, I sort of forgot about being afraid to go to school. I had made a couple of friends by that time and Mother had bought a house right across from the schoolyard. We lived there until I moved away from home after I finished university. Mother told me years later that on the first day of high school (Grade Nine) she was terrified that I wouldn't go without her. I felt bad for her when I found this out because it was the furthest thing from my mind. I walked over a mile to high school every day, and despite being bullied by the boys and a few of the "popular" girls, I loved every minute of high school.

You might think this story is evidence that I "grew out of" my fear of going to school without Mother, and this would be true in my case. But before you get any ideas like applying for the school secretary job for your child's sake, remember that my emetophobia was slowly getting worse and worse, even though I stopped being afraid to walk to school alone. So what Mother did (and inadvertently) did not really help—it just resulted in me getting cleverer about hiding and avoiding what I was afraid of.

ACCOMMODATING OR ENABLING

It's natural to want compassion, understanding, and support when you have emetophobia. You also want to feel safe. All those things are possible without your loved one enabling you, but they may instinctively step in to prevent your anxiety from escalating, help you avoid situations that trigger your fear, or offer you reassurance whenever they feel you need it or whenever you ask them for it. Without realizing, your loved ones may be doing any of these well-meaning actions that are actually enabling you or accommodating the phobia. The problem is that these enabling actions reinforce the phobia rather than help you overcome it.

Enabling means to make something possible; unfortunately, it's the phobia that is made possible, and not your recovery from it. From the enabling actions of others, you learn that avoidance or safety behaviors work to keep your fear at bay, so you tend to rely on not only the enabling by your support person, but on the safety and avoidance behaviors themselves. Over time, this prevents you from learning to sit with a certain amount of anxiety or discomfort, making the phobia even harder to overcome. Supporting you doesn't mean making it easier for you to live *with* your phobia. Support should allow you to recover with ease because you're not alone in it. Support means someone is there with you to encourage your recovery efforts and to help you respond to your anxiety in a healthy way. It doesn't mean keeping you from experiencing any anxiety at all.

"Accommodating" is a word we use to describe how your loved ones behave when you get anxious about something and demand that they change their behavior to "help" you not be so anxious. For example, you may insist that your parents wash their hands many more times than is necessary or normal for them. Or you may insist your partner overcook the chicken. Parents of kids with emetophobia often just want their child to calm down so they do whatever the child wants in order to achieve that end. What they don't realize is that anxiety, while it feels awful, can't harm their child—solidifying a phobia with accommodating behavior certainly will in the long run.

Here are some examples of enabling behaviors.

1. Avoiding restaurants and social gatherings.
2. Providing constant reassurance. It's common for someone with emetophobia to ask, "Do I look pale?" or "Do you think I'm going to be sick?" repeatedly throughout the day. A loving parent, partner, or friend might reassure them every single time: "No, you're fine" or "You're not going to be sick." While this might calm them down in the moment, it teaches them to rely on external reassurance rather than learning to tolerate uncertainty.
3. Preparing special meals or routines. Parents of children with emetophobia might prepare only "safe foods"—bland, low-risk meals that the child believes won't make them sick.
4. Helping someone avoid sick people.
5. Overusing anti-nausea medication or rituals.

The difference between enabling and supporting

It's important to distinguish between enabling someone with emetophobia and supporting them. Support helps them gradually face their fears in a manageable way while enabling allows them to stay in their comfort zone indefinitely.

Enabling behavior	Supportive behavior
Avoiding all restaurants because they're afraid of getting sick	Encouraging them to try a small meal at a quiet restaurant to build confidence
Providing constant reassurance that they won't vomit	Helping them tolerate uncertainty by saying, "I know this feels scary, but you can handle it"
Preparing only "safe foods" that they aren't afraid of	Slowly introducing new foods in a supportive way
Allowing them to skip work or school to avoid germs	Encouraging good hygiene but helping them see that avoiding situations increases their fear
Encouraging overuse of anti-nausea medication or rituals	Helping them recognize when they're using safety behaviors and gently challenging them

How to shift from enabling to supporting

If you've recognized that you've been enabling someone's emetophobia, don't be too hard on yourself. Your intentions have been loving and protective. But now that you understand how fear reinforcement works, you can start shifting toward more supportive behaviors that encourage resilience and recovery. Here's how:

1. Encourage small steps. Instead of pushing someone into an overwhelming situation, help them take small steps. If they avoid eating in restaurants, start with a takeout meal eaten in the car, then progress to sitting inside the restaurant for a few minutes without eating, and eventually work up to a full meal.

2. Reduce reassurance gradually. If they frequently seek reassurance, try responding differently. Instead of saying, "You're fine," say, "You sound anxious—are you able to sit with this feeling for a bit?"

3. Encourage coping skills. Help them develop coping strategies that don't involve avoidance or safety behaviors. Deep breathing, mindfulness, and meditation as well as a healthy diet and exercise are all useful tools to help lead a calmer, more peaceful life overall.

4. Be patient, but stay the course. Understand that they may resist these changes at first. Fear can be overwhelming, and breaking habits of avoidance is difficult. Stay compassionate but consistent. Let them know you're doing this because you care and because you believe in their ability to overcome their fear.

5. Set boundaries for yourself. If you're a parent, partner, or friend of someone with emetophobia, it's essential to set healthy boundaries. You are not responsible for managing their anxiety for them.

How to ask for support

1. First of all, you have to be ready and willing to recover from emetophobia before anyone can support you properly. If you're not ready and willing, then all your loved one can do is take care of themselves. This means they won't be exhausted in trying to "help" you anymore, so at the very least, they'll have more energy for you when you finally decide to get well.

2. If you are on your recovery journey and have been doing the exposure exercises in this book, your loved one can help and support you. You may find that your anxiety has gotten a little worse since you started the exposure exercises. Perhaps you're getting some of the pictures stuck in your mind, or you may be having full-blown panic attacks either as often or more often than usual. The "cure," by the way, for a picture stuck in your head is to go back and look at the picture. I promise you it won't be as bad as it is in your head. This is just another way for your lizard brain to convince you to avoid all this stuff so it won't kill you. Remember: it won't kill you.

3. Ask your support person to stop enabling or accommodating you. The main way that loved ones enable is by offering reassurance that you won't be sick. However, they don't know if you'll be sick or not, so they're just responding to you, saying what you want to hear. This is pretty ridiculous if you think about it. Be sure to tell your loved one that no matter how much you beg, or how angry you get, not to reassure you. Because you really need the help getting over the phobia—not keeping it stuck.

4. Give the following script to your support person and let them know that this is exactly the way you want to be supported. Promise them that you will try your best not to get angry or upset when they do exactly as you have asked and keep this promise! If you don't feel you can make this promise and keep it, then say something like this:

Here is a script that I want you to use to support me in my emetophobia recovery. I can't promise that I won't get unreasonable at some point and demand that you go back to your old way of supporting me, but please don't give in to that demand. Just stay the course and know that I love you.

Script for support people

1. Do an internal check that *you* are calm! Nothing is happening to you, and no matter how anxious your loved one gets, no harm will come to them.
2. Ask, "What number are you at, 0–10?"
3. Then ask, "Can you tolerate that number without doing anything to try to change or lower it?
4. If YES, then say, "Okay, good. I'm right here with you."
5. If NO, then say, "Okay, then let's breathe together and try to bring the number down."
   a. Face your loved one and hold both their hands.
   b. Establish eye contact with them—insist they look at you.
   c. Breathe slowly, without saying anything more.
   d. If they can't breathe as slowly as you, then breathe normally. Eventually their breathing will slow to a normal level.

   e. Now begin again with "What number are you at now?" and "Can you tolerate that number?"
6. Repeat this sequence until your loved one's anxiety number is low enough that they can tolerate it.

EXERCISE 1: Exposure—Pictures of people after they vomit

It's time now to use the QR code below to look at pictures of people *after* they vomit and then to look at pictures of vomit itself with no people in the picture. Once you can do all these exposures with no anxiety, you should be able to walk by vomit on the street without getting overly upset or doing a bunch of safety behaviors afterward, like throwing out your shoes. This is a huge step forward!

https://emetophobiahelp.org/figure-4-1-people-after-vomiting/

Take a week to look at these pictures and those at QR code below. Stare at the pictures until you feel no anxiety. You may even be bored with them. Read over Chapters Two to Four this week as well, before you go on to Chapter Five.

https://emetophobiahelp.org/figure-4-2-just-vomit/

SUMMARY

- Recovering from emetophobia is much easier with a strong support network.
- Support is crucial, but it must be done in a way that encourages recovery rather than reinforcing the fear.
- Well-meaning family members and partners may unknowingly reinforce the phobia by enabling or accommodating safety behaviors.
- Examples of enabling include avoiding restaurants and social gatherings, giving constant reassurance, preparing only "safe" foods, helping the person avoid sick people, and allowing overuse of anti-nausea medication or rituals.
- To shift from enabling to support, loved ones should encourage small steps of exposure, gradually reduce reassurance, help the person develop healthy coping strategies, and set boundaries when needed. Consistency is essential.
- I provide a support script for loved ones to follow. It includes staying calm, asking about anxiety levels, encouraging tolerance when possible, and assisting with slow breathing if necessary. The goal is to help the person sit with anxiety rather than fight it, gradually training their brain that there is no danger.
- The chapter concludes with an exposure exercise, looking at pictures of people who have vomited and pictures of vomit alone.

Chapter Five

EATING

I was glad to go to university in my late teens as it meant I didn't have to answer to anyone, especially Mother, anymore. If I didn't want to do something, I wouldn't, and if I wanted to leave, I could leave. Little did I know as I drove off in my 1970 Datsun Cherry 2-door Deluxe that this new freedom would almost cost me my life.

The closest university was about 150 km from my home, so that's the one I chose. When I signed up for a roommate I filled out the questionnaire to ensure I got the most strait-laced, boring roommate possible, because to me that meant she would never party, get drunk, or take drugs and vomit. I got my wish. She was a "total square," as we used to say.

One of the most common problems with having a vomiting phobia is eating. I started out as a child just being "picky," which is such a judgmental label—as though we have some choice in the matter and just like to irritate people with our list of foods that don't make us gag. Mother used to throw her hands up in despair over what I would and would not eat. She had no idea what I was thinking as a kid: *Vegetables are too hard to digest. Meat might not be cooked. Fruit is too acidic. Rice can go rancid.* It kind of left potatoes and pasta with butter, bananas, milk, Digestives, and a few things that came in a package or can like chicken soup. Mother was on my case constantly over my eating. She didn't just encourage me or coach me or plead with me to eat; she was angry that I wouldn't. So to escape her wrath, at least over this issue, I would choke some food down and hide the rest or throw it out when she wasn't looking.

When my roommate left at Christmas to go on a work practicum, I felt like I could finally *not eat* and be left alone about it. Unfortunately, as I only learned many years later, avoiding what you're afraid of makes your phobia worse. By the end of February in my first year, I was down to eating only bananas and milk from the cafeteria. I kept a few Digestives in my room. Then one day, as I sat down to my lunch, I suddenly felt afraid to eat the banana, afraid it would make me sick. The texture seemed gooey and gross, and it made me want to gag. By this time the milk was a bit warm, and after one sip I couldn't look at it again. I stared at the meagre portion of food in front of me and I said to myself, *Anna, you're going to die from this.*

It was not the "You're going to die" panic signal my lizard brain was always sending. This message was coming directly from my neocortex, the part of your brain that differentiates us from the apes. It originated in a place of reason and logic. I was, indeed, going to die if I kept eating like this—or not eating, as the case may be. I could *not* let that happen. One thing I've always been thankful for is that I have always been optimistic. Anxiety I had in spades, but I also had hope. Or maybe I was too much of a determined, strong-assed bitch to just lay down and die. I would figure this out. I had to. So the next day I got up early, skipped all my classes, and set out for the psychology library. Surely there would be something there about a phobia like this. Perhaps I wasn't the only one in the world who had it.

I told the librarian that I had a psychology essay to do on rare phobias. I still couldn't risk telling anyone what my actual phobia was for fear of some hospital room with a lock on the door and maybe a straitjacket and a vomiting guy in a straitjacket beside me. The librarian was eager to help, but the year was 1977, and so the psychology library in its entirety yielded nothing.

Now I know that, before 1983, exactly zero research had been done on this specific phobia of vomiting, or "SPOV," as the researchers call it, so there was nothing to find. I spent about 16 hours in the library that day. I learned that there were a lot of known phobias at the time: heights, spiders, snakes, public speaking, death, disease. I even found a list of rare phobias in one book that listed such things as fear of ducks, bellybuttons, or peanut butter sticking to the roof of your mouth. But vomiting was not on the list. Not a thing about it.

I came to two conclusions that day: first, I was now absolutely sure I was the only person on God's green earth who had this problem; and second, I was going to be single-handedly responsible for figuring a way out of it.

I presumed I was smart enough to solve the problem. I knew that I needed to be alive and weigh more than 85 pounds to get to Phase 2 of my plan for recovery, so Phase 1 had to address the eating. At this point I had no Phase 2, but whatever. First, we eat and get physically stronger. I decided I would just try to go slowly, one bite at a time. But even the thought of it sent me into a tailspin. I couldn't possibly do this alone, and Mother would be no help. I had met some pretty cool friends in the dorm and so I decided to confide in them. Oh, not actually confide in them—that would be ludicrous—but confide to them a fake problem of just not being able to eat. That sounded unusual, but fairly sane. I told them I had no idea why I couldn't eat normal food, but it had been a slow decline, and at this point, I was 85 pounds and about to die. I needed their help as I'd been hiding the amount of food I'd been eating for quite some time, and I didn't trust myself to go down to the cafeteria alone anymore. Those girls were amazing. I can still see their faces, even though I can't for the life of me remember any of their names.

For the first time, I went down to dinner that night with the whole group. A cafeteria worker slapped down a plate of poached sole in butter, Tater Tots, and broccoli with cheese sauce. I didn't take a dessert because, as a kid I had only wanted dessert, and that was the start of what got me into this hot mess. Staring at my plate I could feel the panic rise inside, overtaking my whole body. My mouth and throat instantly dried out and my mind raced with thoughts such as *It will make you sick* or *You're not used to this* or *You can't eat it. You just can't.*

In my hesitation, tears spilled down my cheeks. This was torture. It was inhumane. How could I possibly be expected to do something as awful as eat?

"It's okay, Anna," said the first friend. The rest agreed. Another gently put her arm around me and squeezed my shoulder as I nodded and tried to swallow the nothingness.

"I know."

"Take your time."

I nodded again and she added, "Not too much time or it will get cold."

I laughed with the others as I picked up one piece of fish with my fork. I must have chewed it about a zillion times before swallowing, unaware that five girls had stopped eating and were staring intently at me. When I finally swallowed they all cheered. I think some of them were actual cheerleaders. The din in the cafeteria quieted as others looked over at us briefly.

The second bite was about half of one of the Tater Tots. It tasted good, which was probably the MSG they put in everything back then. Still, I could only eat half. The bite of the broccoli was also good, mixed as it was with a mouthful of cheese and salty tears.

I put my fork down, defeated. "That's all I can eat," I said, which was met with thunderous applause—first from the five girls and then from about 150 other students. The others didn't have a clue what they were applauding, but it was the '70s, so most of them were probably high.

When I got back to my room I threw myself on my bed and sobbed. Sobbed and sobbed and sobbed. The sobbing is hard to explain now. I was proud of myself. I was happy that it had sort of worked. I was sad that I'd wasted so much of my life being afraid. I was afraid that it wouldn't continue to work. I was ashamed of the whole ordeal that night, as I was ashamed of having this phobia. And I was still terrified I would be sick. But to let out all that emotion, I now know, was a good thing. When the sobbing stopped and I thought about the events of that evening, a tiny smile registered on my face. Eating those three little bites was hard, but I did it.

The next day I would eat two bites, at every meal, and three bites the day after. I would continue on this journey of counting bites, and adding one bite per day, for over a year. I had setbacks along the way, such as on days when I didn't feel well or had to do something scary or important. But after the first couple of setbacks, I came to realize that I didn't return to square one: I could pick up where I left off. Twenty-one bites. Twenty-two. By the time I graduated from university, I was eating normally, even though I was still a selective eater, as I am to this day. It's more a texture thing for me: anything slimy and I won't eat it. I can't stand fat, gristle, cartilage, or the slimy skin of fish, to name just a few things.

People with emetophobia may have many different problems with eating, such as:

- Being afraid to eat, in general
- Restricting foods to only those you deem "safe"
- Being afraid of eating "too much"

- Being afraid of eating too quickly
- Being afraid of eating sweets or junk food
- Being afraid of eating anything someone else has touched (such as pizza)
- Being afraid of choking
- Being afraid of not chewing food enough to digest it
- Being afraid to eat in restaurants, or certain restaurants
- Being afraid to eat if someone else cooks
- Overcooking food, especially chicken
- Being afraid to eat before going out
- Being afraid of eating anything past the "best before" date
- Being afraid of eating leftovers
- Being afraid to eat before certain activities
- Stopping eating on any day you feel nauseous or just "off"
- Stopping eating on any day you come into contact with someone who is ill
- Being severely underweight and not being able to eat calories to gain
- Not eating a healthy, balanced diet.

AVOIDANT/RESTRICTIVE FOOD INTAKE DISORDER (ARFID)

ARFID is a fairly new diagnosis. At one time it was only applied to children who, for some reason, were just not interested in food. It is now applied to adults as well. One of the criteria for diagnosis is that the patient has a fear of the *consequences* of eating, such as choking or vomiting. So people with emetophobia who have eating problems fit this diagnosis, although it is still not the primary one. Emetophobia encompasses ARFID just as it encompasses OCD. Sometimes this little fact is important if you're the one being diagnosed because lots of people don't want to think they have more than one mental illness. If you have emetophobia you probably only have one diagnosis: emetophobia.

Treatment for ARFID is much as I described, which I figured out on my own in 1978. The cure is eating, just as it is "gradual exposure." You can't eat all at once and you can't eat just because someone wants you to or expects you to. You must work on this aspect of emetophobia yourself. So this is a good time to ask any support people you have to kindly back off and leave you alone. However, *you* cannot back off and leave the problem alone. Because if you lose too much weight or can't do normal activities, then you're going to end up in a hospital or an eating disorder treatment program. Both places will ultimately put a tube down your nose into your stomach and, if you can't eat your meals, they will pour a bottle or two of Boost® or Ensure® down into your stomach (this is something called a "bolus"). Getting a bolus of food results in stretching your stomach out, which results in the horrible feeling of fullness that you've been avoiding all along. As stopping eating is a medical emergency, caregivers in the hospital will not be concerned about your phobia. So consider this a warning, and don't ignore your lack of eating problem.

AN EATING HIERARCHY

EXERCISE 1: Changing your eating behaviors

Circle all the items in the list of eating behaviors above that apply to you.

Assign each item a number from 1–100, with 1 being the easiest thing to change. Give each item only one number.

You now have a list of items to work on, in order from easiest to most difficult. Start with the easiest item and tackle that first.

You may add these exposures to your calendar and intersperse them with your giving up of safety and avoidance behaviors.

There is only one way around the fear of eating, or through it (unfortunately), and it's to start eating again, to eat more, or to force yourself to eat certain foods or in certain situations you've been avoiding.

You must stretch your stomach very gradually, and I promise you it will stretch. This is as simple as eating just one bite more after you think you're full. This bite will be very difficult. In fact, all the just-one-more bites will be very difficult. Don't give up as life is long and even a couple of years of torturous eating will gain you decades of freedom from fear and enjoyment of food.

When you're ready, go out to eat. If you can only eat a few bites at first, that's okay. Most partners are willing to take up the slack and finish whatever you ordered or take it home to eat the next day.

FURTHER STEPS TO FOOD FREEDOM

EXERCISE 2: Keeping a food diary

Start a food diary (see Appendix 3), writing down everything you currently eat for three days in a row.

Look at the first item on your list from Exercise 1 and begin on day four to change it, one bite at a time.

Compare what you've eaten with the nutritional requirements of your country's food guide.[1] Are you getting enough protein? Vegetables and fruit? Enough calories? Are your foods a variety of different colors, or is everything the color of rice, pasta, fries, and gravy? Don't despair. Every eating problem is overcome one bite at a time.

Review your food diary again after three days. Compare these days to your first three days. You are making progress, so keep going.

Don't let more than two weeks pass before moving to work on the next item on your list.

If these exercises seem to be far too overwhelming to even try, you may like to consider medication for your anxiety, a change in your medication, or an increase in dosage. Lack of eating properly is a serious problem and you should not have to suffer with it.

1 Canada and the USA each have similar *Food Guides*. The UK has *The Eatwell Guide*.

CONTINUING EXPOSURES

EXERCISE 3: Exposure—Pictures of people vomiting

https://emetophobiahelp.org/figure-5-1-people-vomiting/

The pictures found using the QR code above begin easily again, with the first being a rather blurry picture in black and white. The second picture is also in black and white, and the third is the same picture, but in color. Continue slowly through these pictures, only going on to the next one when you feel little to no anxiety. If you feel great relief when you've finished looking at these pictures, you need to go back and repeat the exercise until you don't. Feeling relieved is a reward feeling from your brain, which will further convince you to avoid doing these kind of exposures. Remember also not to try to force your anxiety to go down while looking at the pictures, such as breathing more slowly, relaxing, or telling yourself any soothing or reassuring things (for example, "It's not real" or "You're okay").

SUMMARY

- When I suddenly found myself afraid to eat even a banana, I realized my life was at risk.
- At the time, no books or studies on emetophobia existed, and I believed I was the only one struggling with this fear. Determined to survive, I devised a plan: I would reintroduce food one bite at a time.
- Eating issues are common in emetophobia and can take

many forms. These eating problems often lead to malnutrition and weight loss.

- Some people with emetophobia fit the diagnosis of Avoidant/Restrictive Food Intake Disorder (ARFID), which involves restricting food due to a fear of negative consequences like choking or vomiting.
- Recovery requires structure. Keeping a food diary can track progress and ensure nutritional balance. Even if the process feels overwhelming now, change is possible, one bite at a time.
- Medication may help stabilize your emotions enough for you to begin eating again or doing exposure work.
- The next step in our exposure work was looking at pictures of people vomiting. You have now completed looking at all the pictures!

Chapter Six

ADDRESSING ANXIOUS THOUGHTS

AUTOMATIC NEGATIVE THOUGHTS

You may not realize it, but your mind constantly generates thoughts—thousands upon thousands each day. Some are helpful, some are neutral, and some are unhelpful. The unhelpful ones are what we call automatic negative thoughts, or ANTs (see Figure 6.1). Without invitation, these thoughts pop into your head, often bringing fear, doubt, or self-criticism. They are fast, persistent, and, most importantly, they feel absolutely real—even when they aren't.

ANTs are sneaky. They whisper things like, *What if that bag of groceries is contaminated with norovirus germs? That's going to make you sick!* or *You can't handle this.* They can appear out of nowhere and immediately change how you feel. One moment you're going about your day; the next, a single thought sends you into a spiral of anxiety, shame, or self-doubt.

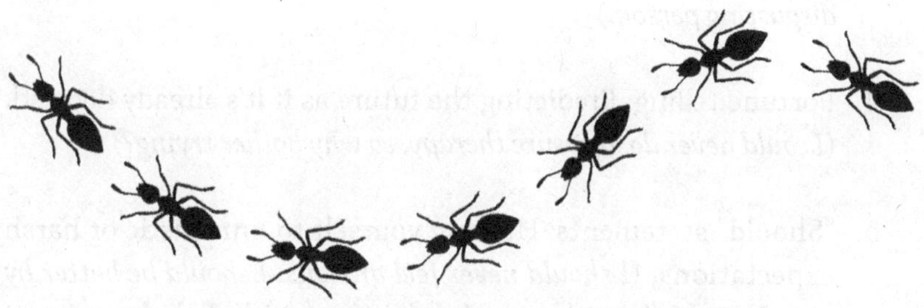

Figure 6.1. ANTs, **A**utomatic **N**egative **T**houghts

This is the sad but sorry truth: as a person with an anxiety disorder, your thoughts cannot be trusted. They're either not true or they lead you down the wrong road and should never be followed. This is also the case if you suffer from depression, in which case your thoughts may be something like *You're not good enough*, *Everyone will hate you* or *You can't handle something like that.*

RECOGNIZING THOSE PESKY ANTS

The first step in changing your relationship with ANTs is recognizing when they show up. Many people don't even realize they're caught in a cycle of negative thinking because it's become so automatic. But once you start paying attention, you'll notice patterns in the types of thoughts you have and the situations that trigger them.

Here are some common types of ANTs:

1. Catastrophizing: Expecting the worst-case scenario, even when there's little or no evidence for it. (*If I get sick, I won't be able to handle it, and my life will fall apart. If I panic, I may have a heart attack or go crazy. I would rather die than vomit.*)

2. Black-and-white thinking: Seeing things as all good or all bad, with no in-between. (*If I make one mistake, I'm a total failure. Even after all that therapy, I'm not better, so it's obviously not possible for anyone to recover.*)

3. Mind reading: Assuming you know what others are thinking, usually in a negative way. (*If I vomit, everyone will think I'm a disgusting person.*)

4. Fortune telling: Predicting the future as if it's already decided. (*I could never do exposure therapy, so why bother trying?*)

5. "Should" statements: Holding yourself to unrealistic or harsh expectations. (*I should never feel anxious. I should be better by now. I should give up because I can't keep up with all the homework.*)

6. "What if" statements: Thoughts about the future. (*What if I'm*

sick? What if that chicken isn't cooked through? What if I touch something that someone sick just touched?)

7. Magical thinking: Superstitious thoughts. (*Last time I vomited I wore an orange shirt, so I can never wear it again. I vomited when I smelled freshly cut grass outside, so now I'm terrified whenever someone cuts the grass.*)

Do any of these sound familiar? If so, you're not alone. Everyone experiences ANTs at some point. The goal isn't to eliminate them completely, because that's impossible. Imagine this for a moment: the president of the United States (pick any president) wearing a pink tutu and a hat with a giant pyramid of fruit on it. He arrives for the State of the Union address dancing down the center aisle of Congress. Do you have a picture of that in your head? This is called a *cognition* or another type of thought. Okay, now I want you to forget that thought. Stop thinking about it. It's not true, and you have no need for this cognition anymore, so just forget it. Impossible, right? And so it is with your ANTs. These anxious thoughts that plague you day in and day out are impossible to get rid of, no matter how hard you try. We need to find a different way to deal with them.

OLD-SCHOOL CBT

When I was trained in CBT (or more specifically, cognitive work) we learned all sorts of tools and ideas about ANTs that therapists are still using today. You may have already run across many of them, either with therapists or from books or articles. The first of these is called *cognitive restructuring*, which involves identifying ANTs, "flawed thinking" or "cognitive distortions," and challenging them. First, you would write down the thought and then answer a series of questions to determine if the thought was true. For example, the magical thought *If I wear an orange shirt again I will vomit* is simply not true. There is no evidence that the shirt caused your vomiting or is in any way related to it. Some ANTs such as *What if that chicken wasn't cooked through and it makes me sick?* could be true, but the thought isn't helpful for your recovery. Many things that people with emetophobia think are true, but not helpful.

Once untrue, flawed, or unhelpful thoughts are identified, we were taught to replace them with more positive thoughts. For example, whenever you think *What if I touched something and then touched my face?* you are meant to "replace" that thought with something like *Vomiting isn't harmful, so it doesn't matter if the chicken makes me sick* or *Normally the worst doesn't happen* or *Vomiting is normal, natural, and neutral* (one of my favorites), or even *"Bring it on—I hope I vomit!"*

When I was going through the last of my ERP therapy, I chose the phrase "You're not in any danger." By that, I didn't mean in danger of vomiting; I meant real life-threatening danger because that's what it felt like to be near anyone who was sick. I wrote this little positive cognition on the back of a business card, and I put it in my pocket when I volunteered at the hospital. I was once asked to sit in on a family meeting with a woman in the end stages of cancer. She was feeling very nauseous and had a plastic bin on her lap. I remember seeing her, and it, when I entered the room along with all the other professionals who were normally on rounds. My heart skipped a beat, and I felt a huge rush of adrenaline. I put my hand into my pocket and felt the card. There was no need to take it out and look at it: I knew exactly what was written on it. Somehow, just feeling the card in my pocket helped me immensely on that day and on many similar days. I liked this cognitive restructuring thing.

I used to use these methods with my patients, often having them fill out forms that I printed where they had to challenge their thoughts, find evidence for their truth, and come up with more logical, rational ones. It worked best with children, I found. Perhaps because their brains are more *plastic*, meaning malleable, reshapable or having the ability to change. I worked with one little kid who was terrified to get on the school bus after someone had been sick on it. One day, at the start of our session, they said, "I got on the bus and went to school every day last week."

"How did you do that?" I asked.

"I just told myself that usually the worst doesn't happen."

I have also employed the phrase "usually the worst doesn't happen" at times when I've been anxious about something other than vomiting. I live on an island in Greater Vancouver at the mouth of the Fraser River, and the best way to travel east is through a tunnel that goes under it. I don't like it. I have visions sometimes of the whole thing collapsing in on me, leading to a watery death. But once I replace that useless thought with *usually the worst doesn't happen*, I'm okay to drive on through the tunnel. Fearing a tunnel collapse, however, is just a fleeting thought, not a phobia, much less a debilitating one like emetophobia.

Before I get too much further, I need to say that just because cognitive restructuring worked for me and a handful of other people, it doesn't mean I endorse it now. In fact, I have found in working with hundreds of people with emetophobia that it is actually a very poor way of helping people with their anxious, repetitive, or obsessive thoughts. It's akin to asking you to forget the image of that president in the tutu and fruit hat. You can change your thought temporarily, or distract yourself by thinking of something else, but you may still be absolutely tormented by the thoughts about vomiting that just go around and around in your head all day, every day.

At one point in the history of psychology, we were told that if we had an intrusive thought, we could snap an elastic band on our wrist. I wonder if these behaviorists spent too much time training animals with cattle prods, because the theory was quickly debunked. I used to just say "Stop!" or "Stop it Anna" or "Stop it Anna—that's not a helpful thought." Doing this is not the same as aversion therapy (snapping an elastic band), but it's a similar idea that again, only worked for a handful of people. As I think back on when I've used this "stop" technique in my life, it has only been with thoughts unrelated to emetophobia. Sometimes I like to beat myself up when someone criticizes my work or my motives. Reminding myself that my self-deprecating thoughts are neither true nor helpful is usually all I need.

In conclusion, all these methods are an old way of doing CBT. None of them work very well for people with emetophobia, perhaps because of emetophobia's close relationship with Obsessive-Compulsive Disorder (OCD)—intrusive or obsessive thoughts cannot be helped, stopped, or eradicated. You cannot make them go away any more than you can forget that image of the president dancing down the aisles of Congress. That's the bad news. The good news is that there is another way of addressing intrusive thoughts, with Acceptance and Commitment Therapy (ACT), known as "second-generation CBT." Before I discuss this new way to handle our thoughts, let's explore emetophobia and OCD.

OBSESSIVE THOUGHTS AND OCD

You probably suffer from an aspect of OCD, which is that once a thought enters your head, you can't seem to get it out. No amount of trying positive cognitions or challenging the thoughts seems to help. Obsessive thoughts are part of OCD, which is shared by all people with emetophobia. As I have mentioned, emetophobia and OCD are somehow related. Because emetophobia is so massively under-researched, we're not sure what the relationship is between it and OCD, but we clinicians know that there is one. I have seen over 300 patients in my clinical practice and educational programs. When they sign up or enroll I ask them to fill out some questionnaires, one of which is the Yale-Brown Obsessive Compulsive Survey (or Y-BOCS). Any score above 7 is indicative of a clinical level of OCD. Not one of my patients or class participants has ever scored in the sub-clinical level. In other words, they all "test positive" for OCD. The QR code below leads to a free online Y-BOCS questionnaire, so you may test yourself if you wish.

https://www.thecalculator.co/health/Yale-Brown-Obsessive-Compulsive-Scale-(Y-BOCS)-Calculator-921.html

There was one study (done by Dr. David Veale and others) that examined the relationship between emetophobia and OCD, which concluded that emetophobia may even be a sub-set of OCD itself.[1] Later Drs. Keyes and Veale speculated that pure OCD was at one end of a continuum and pure emetophobia at the other. Patients with emetophobia fall somewhere along the continuum.[2] This idea and my belief that everyone with emetophobia has OCD are only theories until more scientific research is done.

What matters is that you, as a person with emetophobia, will

1 Veale, D., Hennig, C., and Gledhill, L. (2015) "Is a specific phobia of vomiting part of the obsessive compulsive and related disorders?" *Journal of Obsessive-Compulsive and Related Disorders* 7, 1–6. https://doi.org/10.1016/j.jocrd.2015.08.002

2 Keyes, A., and Veale, D. (2021) *Free Yourself from Emetophobia: A CBT Self-Help Guide for a Fear of Vomiting*. London: Jessica Kingsley Publishers, pp.21–23.

probably show symptoms of OCD that will range from mild to extreme. I once saw a post in my emetophobia Facebook group in which the man described that he was so terrified of germs that he thought about selling his house when he discovered an ER doctor lived down the street and drove on the same roads as he did. He assumed the doctor was spreading germs all over his neighborhood. This is an extreme level of OCD called "OCD, contamination sub-set."

When I was a little kid, I used to have some pretty classic OCD behavior. I "had to" switch the light on-off, on-off, on-OFF, and say that every time I went into my bedroom (it also worked backwards, as in off-on, off-on, off-ON). I also had to walk on the dining room floor tiles a certain way, and if one of my fingers touched a countertop, I had to make sure all five fingers on both hands henceforth touched the countertop. I know I was under seven years old because we lived in Bermuda when I told my dad about this strange behavior that I had—this would have been about 1965. My dad was not a psychologist, remember, but a minister. He said to me, "Those are what we call *habits*, and the only way to break a habit is to just stop doing it." I worshipped my dad and would have stood on my head and drunk root beer if he had suggested it. Because of my trust in him, I completely believed that if I stopped doing these (OCD) behaviors, that nothing bad would happen. So I stopped that very day and never took them up again. Not every child with OCD is so lucky as to have that kind of relationship with their dad that the treatment would be so simple. But to be honest, that *is* the treatment for OCD: stop doing the compulsions or rituals and you'll see that nothing bad happens.

If I get stressed, to this day I will start to clean and tidy stuff up. I'm also a "counter:" I like to count things that do not in any way need to be counted. For example, I used to help my daughter at her bakery by scooping muffin batter into the pans. Each pan held two dozen, so counting the scoops in my head was quite unnecessary, yet I would often catch myself doing it. The OCD brain remains, but I can refrain from doing the compulsions fairly easily. You may not be so lucky, and that's okay. Any compulsions you have or rituals that you perform should be added to your safety behavior hierarchy and calendar, and stopped whenever you feel ready over the next three months. Doing these compulsive behaviors or rituals will not prevent you from vomiting, and you're smart enough to know that, so for most people with mild OCD, giving them up should be feasible.

Some of the obsessive thoughts that people with emetophobia have are those that escalate quickly into full-blown panic. Thoughts that enter your mind as panic-stricken are the worst: *OMG! I put my hand in my mouth without washing it! Now I'll be freaking out for 48 hours! Oh no! Oh no!* If your thought is this panic-stricken from the beginning, then it's more likely to keep repeating over and over. Scanning your body all day long for signs of nausea or stomach upset is another type of obsession. So is scanning people in groups or crowds for anyone who might look ill.

WHEN THOUGHTS DICTATE YOUR BEHAVIOR

The problem if you have obsessive thoughts is that it's a natural conclusion that you will have compulsive behaviors as a result. Those behaviors will be in the form of avoidance or safety behaviors. If you're freaked out that you put your hand in your mouth, for example, you may start taking anti-emetic medicine and keep it up for 48 hours. If your behavior isn't quite that drastic, you may take some ginger or peppermint to "settle your stomach," but you can also do something as extreme, such as stopping eating.

You may not be able to stop thinking your intrusive thoughts, but you can certainly stop acting on them. When I was about 12 years old, Mother decided to take me and her sister Sadie to Prince Edward Island (PEI) to see the sights before heading down south to my grandpa's farm in Nova Scotia for the summer. We ate coleslaw at a restaurant. I normally didn't like it, but this one tasted weirdly sweet. My aunt didn't like it and only had a couple of bites. Mother ate about half of it, but I gobbled the whole thing up. Just about exactly two hours later, the three of us were sick, the severity of said sickness in direct proportion to how much coleslaw we had eaten. My aunt had some mild symptoms, Mother was about half as sick as I was, and I was the sickest. We were in a motel that was up a hill from the office, and as it was about 1970, there was no phone in our room. Don't even get me started on one washroom for the three of us. After a couple of days, Mother and my aunt realized they were still too weak to drive, so as I was younger and healthier, I was appointed to walk down the hill to the office, phone my uncle John on the south shore of Nova Scotia, and somehow walk back up the hill. I remember crawling at one point. Uncle John got into the car with my Uncle Walter and made the five-hour drive to get us and our car. At that time, PEI only had a ferry, not a bridge, which added an extra couple of hours to their ordeal.

After this day, my obsessive thoughts about eating, especially in restaurants, escalated. If I had been an adult, these thoughts may have dictated to me that I never eat out again. But I had a single mother who cracked the whip, so I had no choice in the matter. I do know that I never ordered coleslaw again, and haven't to this day. Never eating a food again that made me sick once certainly isn't necessary, but I share this experience with just about everyone alive. But avoiding all restaurants, and all food in them, all of the time, is completely unnecessary. It seems Mother was right about some things.

ARE INTRUSIVE THOUGHTS JUST YOUR ANXIETY MONSTER?

Many therapists suggest that you think of your anxiety as a "monster"—something external, powerful, and out of your control. As such, they tell you that when you have intrusive thoughts, it's just a monster talking to you and you should tell it to "get lost" in no uncertain terms, cursing at it notwithstanding. I understand as well as anyone that it can feel like a shadowy figure lurking in the background, waiting to strike at any moment. When it shows up, it grips your body and mind, sending waves of fear and panic that feel impossible to stop. But here's what I and many ACT therapists believe: your anxiety is not a monster. It is not an enemy to be fought, nor a curse to be removed. It is a part of you, a protective system that has simply become overactive. Thinking of it as a monster sets up a struggle with your thoughts. Struggling or arguing with your thoughts can seriously inhibit your recovery, mainly because you'll probably be doing it forever.

Anxiety exists for a reason. It evolved as a survival mechanism, designed to keep you safe. Long ago, your ancestors faced real, life-threatening dangers. If they heard a rustle in the bushes, their heart rate soared, their muscles tensed, their bowels loosened, and their bodies flooded with adrenaline, preparing them to flee or fight. This response kept them alive. Today, the world is different. You aren't running from predators, but your brain doesn't always recognize that. Instead, it sounds the alarm when you're faced with a stressful situation—public speaking, an important meeting, a sick child, feelings of nausea, or just the thought that you might be sick. Anxiety isn't trying to destroy you; it's trying to help you. It's just working a little too hard.

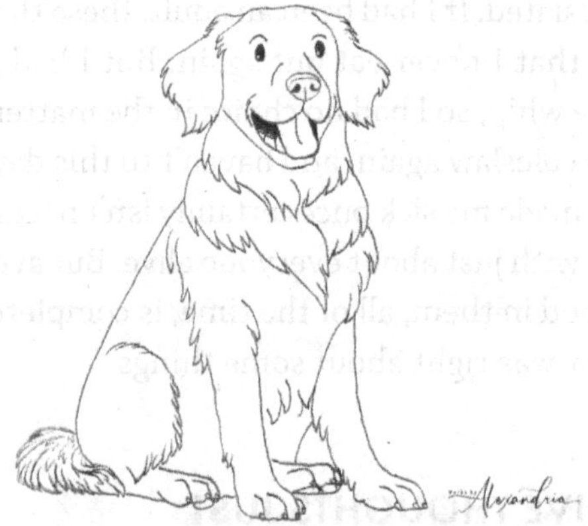

Figure 6.2. Golden Retriever
Source © E. Alexandria Bois 2025

I like to think of my anxiety as a Golden Retriever assistance dog (see Figure 6.2). If you have an assistance dog, it is trained to protect you and warn you of any danger you might encounter. But sometimes even the best assistance dogs make mistakes. I have a friend with an assistance dog who went squirrely trying to get him out of his apartment during a fire drill. My friend had been informed of the drill, but because he was sick in bed that day, he was told he didn't need to participate. Rover did not get the memo, however, and no matter what the man did, the dog wouldn't settle down until the man literally left the apartment in his wheelchair (long after the drill was over) and then went back inside. This story makes sense to us who know how dogs think and why they would act that way. Your anxiety is very much the same, though. Your assistance dog is telling you that you're in danger and need to leave the building, triggering anxiety in your body to prepare you to run, against all common sense. It's a lot of work to put up with a whacko dog for the day or spend hours retraining it, so you end up just following its lead and avoiding what you fear. In other words, *you obey the dog*, instead of the other way around.

WHY THE "MONSTER" METAPHOR IS HARMFUL

When you think of anxiety as a monster, you create an enemy and a conflict. You see it as something that's "out to get you," something to be battled and defeated. But this mindset can backfire. You may have been taught not to fight with your monster, but isn't that even more scary? The more you resist the fight, the stronger your anxiety can seem. Fighting anxiety is like struggling in quicksand; the harder you try to escape, the deeper you sink. Instead of treating your anxious thoughts as an enemy, what if you saw them as just a misguided canine friend? Every good friend—even a human one—can worry too much and jump to conclusions. A human friend can also give you terrible advice, even though at their core they just want to keep you safe. Shifting perspective from thinking of anxiety as a monster to seeing it as a helpful dog can be a game-changer.

Viewing anxiety as a monster can also make you feel helpless, especially on those tough days when the obsessive thoughts just will not quit going around and around in your mind. It may be that you have a very strong personality, so you feel you can fight the monster. But not everyone does. Many people with emetophobia already feel weak, ashamed, helpless, and useless against it.

Seeing anxiety as a monster forces us to engage with it at times, such as "Tell your anxiety monster to get lost." However, you should, if at all possible, leave your anxiety alone and tolerate the way it feels. My friend's assistance dog would eventually stop getting upset at the sound of a fire alarm if it went off all the time, and he would just end up lying down by his owner's feet and going to sleep, saving his protective energy for another day.

A colleague, Canadian clinical psychologist and emetophobia researcher Robert Roopa, whom I interviewed for my podcast, first gave me the idea that seeing your anxiety as a monster is actually a safety behavior. Roopa says, "If you meet the fear with a negative reaction, it gets processed as a safety behavior. You want to approach the fear with a much more neutral emotion."[3]

Giving all that energy to a thought that's a monster no less only encourages it. Building resistance to your anxiety "monster" is giving

3 Christie, A. [Host] (2025) "Is your 'anxiety monster' a safety behaviour? ~ psychologist Robert Roopa." S5E20 [Audio podcast episode], April 18. *Emetophobia Help with Anna Christie* [Audio podcast]. www.buzzsprout.com/1307773

it a lot of attention and energy that will keep you ruminating on it for a great length of time, and that is precisely what you're trying to avoid. Anxiety is not a separate force attacking you; it is a function of your own nervous system. It's your brain's misguided way of trying to protect you, even if it gets things wrong sometimes. When you externalize anxiety—when you label it as a monster—you reinforce the idea that it is bigger and more powerful than you. But it isn't. It lives within you, and because of that, you have the ability to work with it.

News flash! You don't have to eliminate your anxious thoughts (and feelings) to live a fulfilling life. You don't have to be fearless to pursue your dreams. Anxiety might always be there in some form, but it doesn't have to control you or keep you from living life according to your values. All your core values can be done or achieved even if anxious thoughts and feelings are present while you are doing them. If you treat your anxiety more like a Golden Retriever that deserves a pat on the head and a "Thanks, buddy, but I don't need you right now" rather than a horrible monster out to annihilate you, then eventually your anxiety will lie down by the fire and only jump up to warn you if there's an actual threat—a real fire or a person in your house with a gun.

THE ACT APPROACH

Instead of fighting anxious thoughts, consider a new approach: let them be there without struggling, fighting, or arguing with them. Remain neutral toward them. Even though these thoughts may be true (you might get sick), you know for sure that they're not helpful. So don't yell at them to get lost, and don't try to reason with them (have you ever tried to reason with a dog?). Acknowledge their presence. This doesn't mean giving in to them and doing what they tell you, but rather, recognizing that although you can't make them go away, you can rob them of a lot of their power.

Shifting away from the monster narrative allows you to take back control. It empowers you to meet your anxiety with understanding rather than fear. You are not at the mercy of anxiety; you have the strength to live with it with confidence. Your anxiety is not here to ruin your life. It is not a monster lurking in the dark. It is a part of you that just needs a bit of retraining. And the more you learn to work with it, the more power you reclaim over your own life.

Remember "Exercise 1: Establishing your core values" in Chapter Two? If it's been a while, go back and do that exercise again or review what you decided. Noted ACT therapist and author Russ Harris describes our life choices in terms of moving toward or away from our values.[4] For example, if you value work, then working moves you toward that value, while lying on the couch, mindlessly scrolling through TikTok, moves you away. With emetophobia, a choice to get on a plane and travel despite your anxiety is a toward-move, while cancelling the trip because of your anxiety is an away-move.

EXERCISE 1: Addressing intrusive thoughts

Take a few minutes now to write down all your intrusive thoughts. List and number them on a page. Include every anxious thought that has tormented you over the past few months. Remember that all these thoughts are in danger of triggering one of your away-moves.

Even though your anxious, obsessive, or intrusive thoughts may always have to be there, they don't need to have so much power over you. Gaining distance from them is possible, which will rob them of much of their power, but it is a skill that needs to be learned and practiced. Just like tolerating or accepting your anxiety when it hits you, you must practice the skill of detaching ("defusing") from your anxious thoughts when your anxiety is at a low level. An SUD score of 9 or 10, a full-blown panic attack, is not the time when much learning can take place. At lower levels, Harris suggests you try this approach when you are plagued with an obsessive, intrusive thought:

Notice the thought, as though you're seeing it from a distance. Try saying, *I'm having the thought that . . . .*

4 Harris, R. (2022) *The Happiness Trap: How to Stop Struggling and Start Living*. Shambhala, pp.12–25.

To gain even more distance, try: *I notice I'm having the thought that ....*

Now commit to getting on to what you value in life.

Harris also suggests that you try singing your thoughts to the tune of "Happy Birthday," or any other silly tune you can think of. You can also imagine your thought being spoken by a cartoon character in a funny voice. If you try to sing your thoughts or imagine them in a funny voice each time a troubling thought comes to you, you may eventually find that these thoughts have less power over you. That's because you'll begin to see the thoughts for what they really are: just thoughts. They're a bunch of words in your head. They're like a comic book with no pictures, just squares with words in them. Those words are unfairly causing you to do things that don't make sense (away-moves), and they keep your phobia going.

ABIDING

Abiding means "living with," and this is by far the best way to deal with your anxious thoughts. Just let them be there. You may gently remind yourself from time to time that these are just thoughts, but other than that, don't try to address them, argue with them, reason with them, call them a monster, counteract them, or try to make them go away. Resistance is futile, as they say. Practice noticing them as best you can.

Abiding with your thoughts acknowledges that thoughts are just thoughts, not threats. They're just meaningless prattle going on in your head, so they should have no consequence in your life. You know how you can be annoyed by a ticking clock, but eventually, you don't even notice it? That's because you gave it no value, no power. You didn't try to think about its significance; you just ignored it. My house backs on to an elementary school, and sometimes my online patients have to ask me to close the window because the kids at recess are so loud. I've lived here for 25 years, and I don't know when it happened, but at some point I stopped hearing those kids: their screams of glee, their playful laughter. They have no power or consequence in my life, after all. I'm not in charge of them, nor do I even know them, so my brain figured out at some point that I don't need to hear them. I just file away their noise in the "meaningless input" part of my brain. Yet, like the ticking clock, they are still there. I didn't make them go away, as that would be impossible.

Why would you give your nonsensical thoughts about vomiting any more power than your ticking clock or the kids on the playground behind my house? Part of the answer is that you think about vomiting as some huge catastrophic event akin to a terminal cancer diagnosis. But it isn't. It's a big fat nothing. It's normal, natural, and neutral. There's no need to give it any more power than it's worth, which is next to nothing. Your thoughts are an automatic response from your anxiety, not from any part of reality.

The "party" metaphor

Vomiting just doesn't matter, so thoughts about vomiting need not be struggled with, listened to, argued with, or entertained. Another way of looking at this is that you've thrown a huge party with all your friends. Suddenly, a real jerk you didn't invite shows up. You notice them across the room and your heart sinks. This jerk's presence will ruin the party! Your temptation is to go over to them and to try to convince them to leave. You could use all sorts of reasoning, urging, and persuading. But if you do that, you'll be ignoring your other guests and the whole party itself. *You* will be ruining your own party by spending all your time with this jerk. Ignore the jerk. Party on. This metaphor is about obsessive thoughts: the jerk is the thoughts, the party is your life and your core values. Getting on with life is committing to only doing what you truly value. Getting on with something you value helps you to ignore those pesky thoughts. Your values may be lived by doing something as simple as cooking, driving your kids to their sports, or spending time with your cat.

Abiding vs. distraction

Abiding with your thoughts or just leaving them alone and getting on with your life is not the same thing as using distraction as a safety behavior. Distraction means that your anxiety goes up, so you quickly grab your phone and try to play a game, so you forget about the anxiety. It's a thin line, and sometimes we're not sure which we're doing: abiding or distracting. Distraction would be an away-move, doing something fairly useless to try to stop the obsessive thoughts. Getting on with life *notices and acknowledges* the anxious thoughts rather than tries to pretend they don't exist. Distraction is a type of denial where you actually fear the thoughts themselves, so you try to put them out of your mind altogether.

WORDS MATTER

I used to think that vomiting was an absolute nightmare—either if I did it, especially in public, or if someone else did it near me. When I say absolute I really mean *absolute*: the worst nightmare one could possibly ever experience. I would rather have been blown up in a war. I would rather have died.

In 1986, just three years after I had the ERP therapy in Dr. Philips's group, I went to a theological seminary. One of the things I learned there was the importance of the language we use. We were told the first week to divide into two groups and to make a collage of pictures. Our group was given the title "Urban Man" and the other group was given the title "Urban Life." We did not know each other's titles. When the collages were finished, our group with the title "Urban Man" had put together a whole collage of faces that were all men. We didn't even think about cutting any other faces out of the magazines we were given. The other group's collage had men, women, and children. It was rather shocking, especially to me, a feminist who literally burned her bra in the '70s. But the exercise was meant to demonstrate that the words we use have power to influence the way we think.

There is still some discussion today, some 40 years later, about how we can make our language inclusive and the impact that the words we use can have. Our words influence how we think. The words you use to describe vomiting influence your thoughts and, therefore, your feelings. If you continually use phrases like "a horror show," "the most disgusting thing ever," and "my worst nightmare," then you will continue to convince yourself to catastrophize the act of vomiting, which is really nothing more than an uncomfortable inconvenience meant to help your body by ridding it of toxins.

Here are some words and phrases to watch for:

- My worst nightmare
- A living hell
- I am doomed
- Absolutely unbearable
- My biggest fear
- The thing I dread most
- Total loss of control
- A terrifying experience
- Completely horrifying
- I could never cope with it
- 100 percent awful/terrible/horrible/disgusting
- A fate worse than death
- The worst possible thing
- Avoid it at all costs
- A total disaster
- Completely overwhelming
- A catastrophic event
- I can't even think about it
- I would rather die
- I'm afraid if it starts it will never stop.
- So disgusting I could never deal with it.

If you catch yourself saying any of these things, especially out loud, you need to try to stop doing it. This is not the same as trying to stop an intrusive thought, as I've already discussed.

MEDICATION

If you have given all the techniques outlined in this chapter a good ol' college try (for many months or even a year or two) and still you are plagued day in, day out with obsessive thoughts, it may be time to consider medication. There is no need, in the 21st century, to suffer constantly with obsessive thoughts. There are many good anti-obsessional drugs on the market, and more are being developed all the time. Please speak to your doctor, psychiatrist, or other qualified medical practitioner, as they are more in a position to help you with your obsessive thoughts and anxiety levels.

You may already be taking anti-depressants or anti-anxiety meds (which are the same, as it is the same chemical problem in the brain). You may also be in therapy, or you may have already read this book through and done the exercises. If so, and you're still bothered by obsessive thoughts, then perhaps talking with your medical professional about a change in your medication may help. My patients who went on to anti-anxiety meds or changed their meds were often helped to lead calmer, happier lives when they combined medication with our work together. There is no shame in taking these drugs—it's a chemical deficiency in your brain, through no fault of your own. If something were deficient in your pancreas (as with diabetes) or your thyroid, you'd have to have drugs to help you. The brain is just a different organ is all. Having a problem with your brain says nothing about your level of intelligence or your sanity. We've known that since Sigmund Freud, who died in 1939.

EXERCISE 2: Exposure—Watching videos

It's time to watch videos of vomiting, something you probably thought you'd never be able to do. Don't worry—they start with easy ones, and nothing gross. In one way, the videos are easier to watch because the pictures are frozen in time, whereas the videos are over in 2–3 seconds. You can do it! Be sure not to use any safety behaviors while you're watching, such as sipping water, standing up and pacing around, or fidgeting with your hands. Sit on your hands if you have to (use the QR code below).

Take this exercise slowly. Be sure you are almost bored with a video before moving on to the next one. "White-knuckling" through the videos will have the opposite effect you're looking for. Watch them until you can do so calmly. Most of my patients take three or four weeks to get through all these videos, so don't go too quickly. Over that time period you can also practice addressing your thoughts differently.

https://www.youtube.com/
playlist?list=PLnlkxrzYiM_YDc1Ore4ty6vahvh-EtKTW

SUMMARY

- Automatic negative thoughts (ANTs) are problematic for people with anxiety and/or depression.
- There are seven common types of ANTs for people with emetophobia: catastrophizing, black-and-white thinking, mind reading, fortune telling, "should" statements, "what if" statements, and magical or superstitious thinking.
- You imagined the president with a tutu and a hat of fruit on his head dancing down the aisle of Congress, and were then asked to forget this thought, which was impossible.
- Old-school CBT involved identifying untrue or unhelpful thoughts and trying to replace them with more positive thoughts. Snapping an elastic band on your wrist when you had a negative thought was introduced as a technique, but quickly debunked. None of the old-school CBT methods work well for people with emetophobia.
- Obsessive thoughts are part of Obsessive-Compulsive Disorder (OCD), from which everyone with emetophobia suffers at some level.
- Obsessive or intrusive thoughts can dictate your behavior, such as never eating out at a restaurant again.
- Intrusive thoughts are not an anxiety monster; they are more like a misguided assistance dog.
- The "monster" metaphor can be harmful to your recovery. It gives a lot of energy and power to your thoughts. It can even be considered a safety behavior.
- According to the principles of Acceptance and Commitment Therapy (ACT), you don't have to eliminate your intrusive thoughts. Instead, you can allow them to be there without struggle.
- Exercises such as noticing or acknowledging thoughts can be much more helpful.
- Abiding means "living with," and this is the best way to deal with intrusive thoughts. Consider the metaphor of a party

when a jerk shows up. Get on with the party, rather than spend time struggling with the jerk.

- Abiding and distraction are two different things.
- The words and phrases we use to describe vomiting, especially out loud, are important.
- Medication can be helpful for obsessive thoughts.
- You watched videos of vomiting over a two- to three-week period.

Chapter Seven

IN VIVO EXPOSURES

The most common question I get from my patients and the participants in my online classes is, "All this exposure work is about other people vomiting. But my main fear is myself, so how does it help?" It's certainly a valid question, and this chapter and its exercises will help you make that transition from fearing something "out there" to fearing something in your own body.

So long as your anxiety goes up when you're doing the exposure exercises in the previous chapters, then your brain is learning what it needs to learn. Brains have the ability to *generalize*, which means to apply specific learning to other situations. Indeed, these kinds of exposure exercises won't help you 100 percent, but they are heading you in the right direction, especially if you can tolerate anxiety at higher levels than you once thought, like 7 or 8 out of 10.

Conquering your fear of talking about and imagining vomiting, seeing words and pictures, having memories, and watching videos should give you a much-needed boost in confidence and self-worth. If you've been doing all the exercises in the previous chapters, then give yourself a pat on the back or another one of those treats. My favorite thing to do is go out for a chai latte and drink it on a log at the beach near my home. I often sit there and think to myself, *It doesn't get any better than this.* Try it sometime. You deserve it!

Of course there must be more to recovery than doing the online exposure exercises. You should be doing real-life things already, like giving up safety behaviors as well as changing your behaviors around eating. Those have all been plotted on your calendar. How are you doing with those? Don't forget that keeping only *one* safety behavior will mean that your phobia stays with you. Sometimes I've had folks in my classes put a note on their calendars that says something like "I have [an anti-emetic drug] but I'm never giving that up." I'm too nice not to email back "Okay, but just so you know, you're never giving up your phobia either." Work diligently to give up all those safety behaviors!

AVOIDANCE

Avoidance was my go-to safety behavior. Either I pre-emptively avoided places and people where someone might vomit and I couldn't get out, or I ran away like mad if someone said they were ill or if they vomited. I couldn't avoid hospitals because I was a minister and it was my job to visit the sick. Most people in hospital aren't vomiting because there are meds there that prevent it. Nevertheless, the place terrified me. I would dread my hospital visit days and I'd sneak into the patient's room, hoping they were asleep, which they often were. If so, I'd zip back out into the hall and write a little note on my business card saying I didn't want to wake them. If they were awake, I'd go into their room in some sort of dissociative daze. It was like I was swimming through a milkshake with my heart pounding like crazy. I tried to breathe and relax like I had learned in Dr. Philips's group in 1983, but it didn't work. All I wanted to do was get out of there. I always said a prayer with the patient (only God knows how I came up with those), and then made an excuse that I didn't want to tire them out. It usually took until I got out of the hospital and into my car before the fog lifted and, without exception, I would burst into tears. If ever someone had a vomit basin next to them, or even on their table, I would not go into their room or leave immediately. I tried to peek in the most creative ways to see if they had one before the patient saw me. But even if they did see me, I would run for the exits and make up some elaborate story that I had a pager and it had gone off and something had happened at home—I can't remember now, but it was always a whopping lie.

If I didn't get to see someone in the hospital, not only would I feel incredibly guilty about it, but in my small elderly congregations I was often criticized for "not caring." I don't know how many times in my past as a person with emetophobia I was told I was cold, unfeeling, selfish, or uncaring. Sometimes a whole committee would sit me down to tell me this. In reality, I'm a warm and caring person. I care deeply—almost too much sometimes. So this kind of critique killed me inside, as I was reminded of being told the same thing by Mother as a child. The truth is that I was so ashamed of the phobia and so fearful that someone would lock me up and throw away the key that I could not bring myself to tell either Mother or one other single soul. It was easier for me to put up with the fact that everyone thought I was cold and uncaring.

I think the first person I told about my emetophobia was my boyfriend in 1980 when I was 22 years old. He wanted to marry me and have children, so I had to tell him. This news, far from sending him away, didn't deter him in the least, and we've been married now for over 45 years. He promised me he would look after the kids if they were sick, and it didn't occur to me that he might not always be there because he was at work or out of town on business, so I agreed to the whole arrangement at the time. No regrets—three great kids who each chose three lovely mates, and now seven amazing grandchildren.

Of course, I avoided many other things, like riding in the car with anyone but my own family members, running a kids' program without some other grown-ups there to help, getting on any public transit, theaters, the movies, concerts, bars and clubs, and sitting in a chair anywhere at a kids' recital or school performance. You could not possibly drag me onto a plane. Not even kicking and screaming. I would fight you.

Avoiding things pre-emptively confused Mother and my sister. I remember once when I was about 10 years old going to visit my sister and her husband in Toronto. They wanted to take me downtown the next morning to the Santa Claus parade. In 1968 this would have been a huge thrill for any small-town kid like me. I refused to go because I overheard Mother and my sister talking the night before about how we'd have to go on the subway to get there. A subway train, once it started moving, would be a situation where you could not get out if someone was sick. So, just like an airplane, I could not possibly be coaxed into it. However, there was no way I would tell them why—I just said I didn't want to go. Mother was used to me not wanting to do just about anything, but my sister and her husband were confused, and even a bit angry. In the end, I got to stay in the apartment and watch cartoons on their TV, which had multiple channels—at home, we just had the one channel. There were cartoons on my sister's TV that I didn't even know existed, like *Archie*, which was my favorite comic book. I was thrilled to watch those cartoons—it's one of my fondest childhood memories, seeing those comic book characters come alive on the screen. Did I miss out on fun stuff because I was phobic? Maybe. But *Archie* trumped Santa in my book.

The only way out of avoidance is to approach the things you're afraid of, slowly. This may not be possible logistically for you, but that's okay. If you avoid sick people, it's hard to orchestrate an exposure around that, but hopefully, one will come your way at the exact right time and not before.

You also may not be able to approach what you've been avoiding because it's just too scary for you. I remember this. One of my therapists told me to go sit in a hospital ER because people vomit there all the time. The very idea of this completely overwhelmed me, and I told him so. He informed me that when I was ready to face my fears to give him a call. Then he wrote a report to my GP saying I was "non-compliant" with therapy. But the truth was that this was like telling someone at the bottom of the ladder to just jump up to the top rung. Impossible. There had to be a way to break this down into smaller steps.

If you avoid amusement parks, movie theaters, or concerts, for example—or even going out of the house—it won't help you to just force yourself to do these things. You will probably "white-knuckle" it all the way through your time there. This means you'll just be afraid, hoping and praying nothing happens. Remember that the problem with this approach is that once you're home again you'll feel a tremendous sense of relief, which is a reward in the brain. If you cannot figure out a way to slowly approach what you've been avoiding and be able to be calm and happy while there, then don't just "white-knuckle" it. It's better not to go at all until you can go and be calm. Eventually, you will have more confidence in what you once considered a "dangerous" place. We will get to that later.

Here are a few examples of things people with emetophobia may avoid:

1. Travelling by air or sea
2. Amusement parks and rides
3. Bars and parties where people may drink too much
4. Schools, daycare, and nursing homes, where people are often sick

5. Getting pregnant
6. Crowded places like parades, theaters, and cinemas
7. Kids' concerts or parties, soft play, jungle gyms
8. Family gatherings
9. Driving or riding in the car with someone else
10. Medical procedures such as an endoscopy, barium swallow, colonoscopy, elective surgery
11. Caring for sick children or a partner
12. Homes where people have been sick recently, sick people, and hospitals.

These "top 12" avoidance behaviors often relate to your goals in Chapter One. So let's look at each one individually, and see how we might set up an exercise to help you overcome these avoidances.

1. Travel

It's not easy to arrange travel if you have nowhere in particular to go or you can't afford to just frivolously book a trip somewhere for the sake of an exposure. You may be simply putting off a trip or a cruise, in which case, the exercise would be to book it about three to four months in advance, knowing that by the time you get to it, you will be much calmer because you will have worked through the exercises in this book.

I never used to travel when I had emetophobia as an adult. Airplanes terrified me. I wasn't so worried about the plane crashing; I was worried I'd be sat beside someone who was vomiting, or the turbulence would make me sick myself. Eventually, our daughter moved from Canada to Germany to join a ballet company. After all the years of watching her, encouraging her, being a shoulder for her tears, and paying for hundreds of pairs of ballet shoes, there was no way I was going to miss her first performance as a professional. In fact, I booked tickets for two nights in a row, because I knew that the first night I'd just be watching her and crying through the whole thing. This turned out to be true, so luckily the next night I was able to watch the ballet.

We booked flights about four months in advance, so I knew I had to practice my exposure exercises diligently to be able to go. At least I'd be going with my husband, and he was kind enough to book us in first class, so I only had to sit next to him and no one else. I still took Ativan for the flight and slept through most of it. On the way back

I only took half the amount of Ativan, and I got through the flight okay. Then I did something very courageous: I let my name stand for a national committee for our church that met three times a year in Toronto, a five-hour flight from my home in Vancouver. I would be sitting on the committee for three years, so that was a lot of flying, and I had to do it alone. I cried before the first flight and took Ativan which made me too groggy the next day for the meeting. Long story short, I was finally able to travel to Toronto, Montreal, and even Halifax for these meetings, alone, and without any medication. It's all about the practice, and mustering up a sense of determination. Eventually, I enjoyed these flights—meeting new people, and even the airline food. I also looked forward to seeing my friends and colleagues each time, which gave me a sense of "reward" for doing the task.

You may not be able to arrange something like this to address your fear of flying, which is okay because we can approach your fear from another angle. But if you have to fly or take a cruise ship, remember that literally millions of people do this every year, and almost never if they're ill.

If you don't have the money or a reason to take a flight, you can simulate the exposure by riding on a bus or subway. Although the bus will make more stops than an airplane, when the bus is going you are still "trapped," which is the same feeling people with emetophobia worry about feeling on airplanes. Sit next to the window on the bus during rush hour when someone will sit beside you and many people will crowd in, standing. Don't use any safety behaviors. If you have to get off the bus (retreat) that's fine, *so long as you get back on*. Don't just go home or you'll feel wonderful relief at *not* being on the bus and this will put you backwards in your recovery. Try to ride the bus until you're calm and get off when you're calm if possible.

You can "retreat" from riding public transit by getting off at a stop. Retreating is to *temporarily* avoid the situation, which is, of course, a safety behavior. If you retreat, only stay away until you're calm enough to try again. You'll be surprised at how much easier the exercise will be a second time.

2. Amusement parks and rides

It may not be possible to raise kids nowadays without feeling the need to take them to an amusement park or even the local county fair with all the rides and terrible junk food that kids just love. Even if you don't have kids, your partner and/or your friends may like to go and will want you to go with them. The very idea of going may terrify you, even if you don't go on any rides. Once I was over my emetophobia, at our local farm expo I decided to try one of those rides where you fall to your death and then are miraculously saved with a huge splash of water. I'm happy to report that even though I wasn't afraid on the ride, I didn't like it, so I don't plan on ever going again. Rides just don't thrill me.

Again, plan to go some time in the future and book it into your calendar. If it's a local affair (which I would suggest, at first), then tell your partner you are willing to go on a certain date and have them support you by holding you to that date. If you see someone sick at an amusement park, remember that you have seen people vomit on video now and it's really no different. Sick people don't go to amusement parks, so in a way it's a good in vivo or "real-life" exposure if you do see someone.

3. Bars and parties

Write in your safety behaviors calendar (Exercise 2, Chapter Three) a date when you're willing to go to a bar or a party where alcohol is served. This will be an easier exposure than going where someone may be actually sick, because drunk vomiting isn't contagious anyway. You may find that you enjoy yourself. Try not to "white-knuckle" your way through the party so that you feel better once you leave. This feeling better, remember, is a real reward to your brain, and thus your brain will encourage you not to go again because leaving feels so good. The trick is to feel good while you're there!

4. Schools, daycare, and nursing homes

If you don't have a child in school or daycare, or a parent in a nursing home, then going to one may be more difficult to orchestrate. Nursing homes may be your best bet to volunteer some hours as they would love to have you. Read to patients who can no longer see or offer to help with feeding at mealtimes. Drop an email to a few nursing homes near your home and see what happens. You may be surprised at the joy and satisfaction you get from volunteering with this community of people.

If you do have kids in school, you can also volunteer there, even for an hour a week. Perhaps help in the library, with hot lunch programs, or help kids to read. Again, you may be shocked at how much fun it is and how much satisfaction you get out of it.

5. Getting pregnant

If getting pregnant is one of your goals, then there isn't much you can do to prepare yourself for it. I used the Nike philosophy *Just Do It*, and I didn't renew my birth control prescription. I was pretty surprised that I found myself pregnant two weeks later. I guess I was brave enough at the time to just throw caution to the wind. I really wanted a baby, and my desire for one was stronger, at least that day, than my fear. Besides, once I got pregnant I was pretty much stuck with the decision. I have never looked back and never regretted it for one minute. I love my children more than life itself, and all my patients, people in my classes, and thousands online who finally get pregnant say they feel the same way.

Being pregnant in the '80s was another "no internet blessing" because I only factored in that Mother and my sister never got morning sickness. I had none with our second child, but with the third, I was nauseous for the whole nine months. It wasn't great, for sure, but that little girl has been worth every miserable moment, and she's just turning 40 this year.

What I'm trying to say is that the *reward* must be greater than the *cost* for you to throw caution to the wind and get pregnant. Nothing will prepare you for it, but the more you overcome your emetophobia and get to the place of "it doesn't matter if I vomit," the more easily you can make this decision.

6. Crowded places

It's actually easy to add this one to your safety behaviors calendar. Figure out where it fits in terms of how easy an exposure it will be to go to the movies, grab some popcorn and soda pop, and sit in the *middle seat* of the row. So that's a few things. If you've been too afraid to even go to the movies, then it's okay to sit at the end of the row the first time. But be sure to schedule a time when you'll sit in the middle. If it's a concert, a sporting event, or a theater production where seats are assigned, then book yourself the middle seat so you can't chicken out at the last minute. Be sure not to "white-knuckle" your way through the event or the exposure will be useless. Be calm and enjoy it. The first time I sat in the middle seat in the middle row of the theater I thought to myself, *Wow, you really can see better from here!*

7. Kids' concerts or parties, soft play, jungle gyms

Any activity involving a lot of kids together, indoors, particularly in winter, will be difficult for someone with emetophobia. Your thoughts may run away with you and your anxiety may rise. For the sake of your own children, don't refuse invitations for them to participate in such events. Go to their concert. Volunteer to help with every birthday party. Book into your calendar a day that you'll take them to soft play or an indoor gym. Watch the glee on their little faces and their body language when they come racing over to you or yell "Watch me, dad!" Try to take your vibe off them, and not from all the germs you imagine are rampant in the venue. Kids have immune systems and can handle a lot of germs without catching everything. Wash their hands at the end, but don't slather hand sanitizer on them because no one else will be doing that, and your goal is to be "normal" like everyone else.

8. Family gatherings

Special occasions such as Passover, Eid, Thanksgiving, or family birthdays are often difficult for people with emetophobia, especially if they have a big family. Thanksgiving and Christmas in particular (in the northern hemisphere) occur in the winter or autumn, when cold and flu season is at its highest level. Weddings and special birthday parties can fall at any time of the year, but normally all family members are expected to be in attendance. So if you discover that some cousins or other relatives have been ill with vomiting, then attending such affairs may seem incredibly daunting. There is no way to set this up as an exposure exercise except to wait long enough for it to happen. After you have gone through all your other exposures and given up safety behaviors you may be doing fairly well, so the temptation may be to skip the event and call in your regrets. Try not to do that, of course, is my advice.

I was lucky, or perhaps unlucky enough, not to be near any family members when my kids were growing up, so all special occasions were just the five of us anyway. But now, all three of my kids have spouses and two or three kids of their own, so my immediate family has grown to 15. My sister, who lives five minutes from me, adds another six now for a total of 21, if everyone is available—that's quite a crowd and they're not always well. I've learned not to ask, and if anyone offers the information, I just say to myself (after a bit of an initial "jolt"), *Oh well, if we catch it we catch it. It doesn't matter.* This is what you're aiming for.

You can easily schedule a family gathering; if no one offers to host it, then you host. Try not to be angry if someone shows up who says their kid was vomiting the day before but they're okay now. "Normal" people (people without emetophobia) are usually happy to hear that the child is okay today and glad everyone could come. It's not normal behavior to expect them to stay home, or to be upset that they didn't. Remember that if you want to *be* normal you must *act* normal.

9. Driving or riding in the car

Some people with emetophobia also have a fear of driving, even if they're the only one in the car. Fear of driving is a phobia in and of itself, which often stems from the fear of getting into a car accident or of hurting someone else, such as a pedestrian. With emetophobia, it's usually more about being far away from home, as they fear vomiting more if they're not at home. Nevertheless, the fix is the same and it is gradual exposure. If you fear driving or being away from home the treatment is to gradually drive further and further from home. Remember how important it is to be calm and happy that you are far from home. Otherwise, you fall into "white-knuckling" it and it will be a huge reward to your brain when you return home. This won't help you, no matter how many times you take a drive or how far you get from home. So try to set up a nice reward for yourself when you drive a certain distance. Perhaps there's a nice coffee shop, a store you'd like to browse in, or a friend you'd like to see. Whatever it is, it has to be enough of a reward just to make it there, and best if it's even a disappointment that you have to leave and go home. You can always combine exposures such as driving to a movie theater and seeing a film you've been wanting to see.

I, like many other people with emetophobia, really feared riding in a car that someone else was driving who was not a family member. This is amazing considering I taught three teenagers to drive and my son-in-law to drive a stick shift. You'd think that would be nerve-wracking enough. But for me, it was always about someone vomiting in my car or whatever car I was riding in. Like many other people with emetophobia,

I think I overestimated how common motion sickness is. I had ridden in the back of a car halfway across Canada every summer from age nine to sixteen, so I knew full well that I didn't get carsick. It never even occurred to me.

I recall one summer when Mother, Aunt Sadie and I crossed the Bay of Fundy on a ferry. The Bay of Fundy is notorious for huge tides and very rough seas. We had a stateroom with a little table and chairs, bunk beds, and a washroom. When we got on board Mother ordered a salad, Aunt Sadie a ham sandwich, and I ordered a piece of apple pie. Once the voyage started, the rocking of the boat put me off to sleep in the bunk beds. It was about a four-hour ride across. Unbeknownst to me, Mother and Aunt Sadie had been terribly seasick the whole time I was asleep. When I woke up they were still green around the gills, but I was fine. Mother didn't want to say anything about the seasickness because she knew instinctively that it would upset me, so she just smiled and said they weren't hungry, and I could eat whatever I wanted. I ate the salad, the ham sandwich, and the apple pie. Essentially, I don't get motion sickness—experience has taught me this—and again, there were no social media posts about motion sickness to contradict my view. I had no way of gaining any information at all about seasickness, altitude sickness, or morning sickness, except from my own experience.

A huge number of people with emetophobia with whom I work are terrified that they will get carsick, even if they never have before. They often tell me, confidently, "I get motion sick." I wondered about this phenomenon enough that when I had an appointment with an ENT (ear, nose, and throat) doctor for an unrelated matter I asked her about it. She assured me in no uncertain terms that if someone didn't get carsick, as in vomited in the car when they were children, then it wouldn't just magically appear in their adulthood. Carsickness begins when kids are around two years old or even a little younger. The motion of the car disturbs the fluid inside their inner ear, enough that it triggers one of the vomiting centers in the brain. Motion sickness can get better with age, the doctor assured me, but not worse. When I tell this to my emetophobia patients or class participants, they seem to accept it. It's like they really have known all along that they don't get motion sick; it's just anxiety. Anxiety, as you know by now, causes nausea. Real nausea, not imaginary nausea. When you get anxious your digestion slows or stops and this makes you nauseous. Plus most people with emetophobia fear that anxiety itself will make them vomit, even if it never has before.

My fear of driving in cars was always that one of my kids would vomit. We came close several times. I once drove all three kids home from the dentist and my youngest, about age five, said she was going to be sick (probably from swallowing the fluoride they had in those days). I pulled the car over and got out with her, but she didn't get sick. I'm pretty sure she could stop herself from vomiting just so I wouldn't freak out. We jumped back in the car, and while I managed to get her into her car seat, I forgot to do up my seatbelt. I learned later how much this got to my son (age 15 at the time), as I was also driving ridiculously and dangerously fast to get home as speedily as possible. We made it home and into the house before she got sick, the poor little thing. She's 40 years old now and still can't tolerate fluoride or dental cleaning without becoming anxious about it. I blame myself for that, but at least she didn't develop emetophobia.

Another time we were coming home from a baseball tournament in the interior of British Columbia, where temperatures skyrocket in the summer. One town reaches close to 50°C, which is thought to be "unlivable." So it was hot, and our car's air conditioning couldn't keep up, and the same daughter got quite overheated and nauseous. We stopped the car and let her cool off inside a gas station while I tried to calm down outside in the heat. Somehow we managed to get home thanks to the fact I had Valium as a "rescue medication" that I'd never taken before, but it worked and got me home.

The worst story I have about my emetophobia and driving was our trip to Disneyland when the youngest kids were 13 and 11. Our 13-year-old had been invited with her jazz company to dance at Disneyland, and we were given free tickets for the day as well as the kids, and their siblings were given a guided tour of the "underground" of Disneyland. The dance moms organized a chartered flight, hotels, and food. I had emetophobia so bad that I was terrified to fly. As we raised our kids on a shoestring budget, living paycheck to paycheck, I knew that this would be their only chance to go to Disneyland, but we had to drive, because I was too afraid that one of them, or another person, would be sick on the plane.

It was a long trip from Vancouver to LA, through the hot desert and such, but I organized activities, and we sang Disney songs all the way there. Once we arrived, we met up with the group and had a great time. But on the way home we decided to drive the "scenic route" through the state of Oregon. I was driving around a very curvy road. We had a Toyota minivan with two seats in the middle and three in the back. Due to my emetophobia, I insisted the two girls always sit in the very back with my youngest (the one with the weak stomach) sitting behind the middle seat so I couldn't even see her. I always put a garbage can between them. Sure enough, at one point I heard a tiny little cough. I looked in the rearview mirror and asked what was up. Katie said, "Lizzie threw up." I slammed on the brakes and pulled over. "In the garbage can!" she added excitedly as if that would make it all okay. It didn't.

There was barely a shoulder on the side of the road as the edge of the road went straight up. I ran up that hill, sat down, and freaked out like never before. "I want my dad," I said, over and over. My husband was sitting beside me, trying to calm me down. Dad had died in 1968, close to 30 years before. I knew this to be true, but I couldn't stop saying it anyway: "I want my dad." It eventually gave me a lot of insight into the root of my phobia, even though that didn't make a whit of a difference in the treatment of it, much less at that moment.

I refused to get back in the car for what seemed like an inordinate amount of time. The thing about panic attacks or anxiety that's at its worst level possible is that the anxiety has nowhere to go but down. The worst has now happened, and I came to the realization that flying there and back was probably the safer version of the trip, so I was greatly embarrassed by the whole thing. Finally, I got back in the car, but not before telling Elizabeth that my behavior was absolutely not her fault and that she couldn't help being sick. It turned out it was the swingy roads that made her sick, so we stopped for the night as soon as possible. Somehow I pulled myself together, and we continued on our trip home on the eight-lane highway.

Needless to say, I never liked car trips, and even after being successfully treated for the emetophobia I still had the urge to avoid them, especially with kids in cars. Thankfully, in about 2015, my grandson vomited in the car while I was driving 50 km to his mother's bakery. I calmly pulled over at a gas station and convenience store so my daughter could get some paper towels and things to clean him up. It was like night and day. Recovery is always the answer to approaching what we have avoided.

It's easy to schedule exposures for yourself around driving with others, but it's not so easy not to feel relief when you get home. Again, try to make the journey fun so that you can experience a state of calm and happiness while you are out. This may take many, many repeats of the exposure. But what is your alternative? When they say recovery is hard work, they mean it.

10. Medical procedures

Doctor
Dentist
Chiropractor
Optometrist
Therapist
Physio
Blood test
Medical test

Figure 7.1. Appointments I need to make

The only way to get over your fear of having any given medical procedure is to book the procedure. You can let your doctor know about your fear (there is nothing to be ashamed of) so perhaps you can be sedated or given anti-emetics or whatever you believe may help you. Are these not safety behaviors, you may well ask? Yes, they are, but I give a "pass" to people who need a medical procedure because getting the procedure is more important than overcoming your fear of it right now.

I have cancelled several procedures in the past. One was a cystoscopy due to UTIs (urinary tract infections) I had in my 20s, another was an MRI of my hip after a car accident, and later an endoscopy where they look down into your stomach. It was only after I was recovered that I knew I had to start showing up to these appointments. I started by taking Ativan for them and asking for anti-emetics, but eventually, I was able to do them without either. Ativan and other tranquillizers are benzodiazepines and therefore highly addictive. They are fine to take for occasional use such as flying, going to the dentist, or before a procedure with the understanding that you are working toward eradicating your fear altogether so the day will come when you no longer need them. Medical tests and procedures are normally important for your health, and this includes dental work, so start calling or emailing and making your appointments for some time over the next three to four months (see Figure 7.1).

11. Caring for sick children or a partner

Generally speaking, your partner doesn't need any "help" if they are vomiting. Normally fit and well adults who aren't drinking or taking drugs can vomit just fine on their own, and most of them don't want anyone around while they do it anyway. If your partner or friend has drunk too much or taken a drug that is making them sick, they may need your help, though. If the person is passed out they need to be rolled onto their side in what is called the "recovery position." It's probably safest to call an ambulance for anyone who is unconscious or non-responsive. Most people with emetophobia aren't afraid to help people who are vomiting from something that isn't contagious. I would not have cared what the reason was—I ran away from anyone vomiting or about to vomit for any reason.

Children are another story, and even though your partner may care for them when they're sick, they often want you anyway. So many of my patients tell me they feel like "terrible mothers," or they're ashamed to admit that they are more afraid of catching a virus from a child than of the child being sick themselves. You are not a terrible mother or father if you're afraid of your child when they're sick. You have an anxiety disorder, and you're reading this book to try to overcome it.

You can't help the fact that you have the disorder any more than you could help the fact you have diabetes, gallstones, or appendicitis. If you're a "terrible mother" or a "terrible father" reading this, then I take the all-time prize.

I was so scared of my own kids when they were sick that I would run away from them. If my husband was home, I would hide in our basement with the door locked and fingers plugging my ears. For days. I wouldn't eat or drink, and I would definitely not come upstairs. I've had patients who took up residence in a suite in their basement meant to be rented out but saved just for this occasion, and others who moved out of the house to their parents, or even to a hotel. We had no parents nearby and no money for hotels, so plugging my ears in the basement was all I could do. Even when the kids were toddlers, if they vomited, let's say, in the kitchen, I would run away, but then go back a few seconds later. I'd pick the kid up and plunk them in the bathtub or in their crib. After a phone call to my husband to beg him to come home from work, I would clean up the kitchen and stand outside the door of the washroom or bedroom and peek around the corner every once in a while to make sure the child was still living and breathing. Once my husband got home, I would fall apart and escape to the basement.

Being able to care for their kids when they're sick is the number one goal my patients have. This is something that some avoid, as I did, although surprisingly most of them *are* able to look after their own kids because a parent's instinct takes over and overrides the fear. I never had this instinct, probably due to my childhood trauma, losing my primary caregiver (my father) at the age of nine and Mother being an angry and emotionally abusive parent. I have it now, for my grandchildren. I could easily look after them when they're sick, and even though I might still get a little jolt of fear or adrenaline, my love for them would override that. My kids missed out on this from me, but I still have a great relationship with each of them as they do with each other.

You can't plan for exposures around caring for sick kids. But you can stop avoiding places to take them so that they may be more likely to be sick. Yes, you heard that right. Lean into the fear and take your kids to those germy theme parks and jungle gyms. Let them play and feed them hot dogs later before they wash their hands. Soon enough, your wish for an exposure exercise around caring for sick children will probably come true. If it doesn't, that's fine too.

12. Sick people

Usually, the top of everyone's hierarchy is "being around sick people," and by sick, we mean vomiting. Perhaps it's letting your child play at the neighbor's house when they have all recently had norovirus. Perhaps it's inviting someone to your own home who you know has been sick, even if you don't know the cause. One of my patients once asked me if I thought it was okay to eat some cookies that were dropped off by a neighbor because they had all been sick a few weeks before. Visiting loved ones in a hospital or accompanying someone to the ER can be particularly stressful. How do we plan for this kind of exposure?

It is difficult to plan but not impossible. Depending on what country you live in, it may be possible to plan to sit in the ER waiting room for a few hours reading a book. That would not be possible where I live because you have to check in at the door so you can be triaged. But your country or state might not pay such close attention to who is in their waiting room. If it's not possible to just walk in and sit, you will need some help. If you have any friends who are doctors or nurses, ask if they can arrange this for you.

My final step in exposure therapy was to volunteer at the hospital. I was very fortunate that I was trained as a hospital chaplain in theological college, so I made an appointment with the chaplain in residence and explained to him that I would like to spend two weeks (my vacation time) in the hospital as a volunteer chaplain under his supervision. I also told him that I was trying to overcome a phobia of people vomiting. He was very kind and excited about having my help for a couple of weeks. He assigned me to three floors and the ER, specifically, medical, pediatrics, and palliative care. I was taken for an ID badge that read "Spiritual Care" and sent on my way to introduce myself to the supervising nurses, social workers, and ward clerks. This was a time before privacy laws, so I was allowed access to patient charts, and I went looking specifically for people who may be vomiting. I had a nurse friend on the medical ward, one in surgical recovery, and another on pediatrics.

My time began with one nurse friend kindly arranging for me to be present in the recovery room after surgeries, although she said that with the great drugs they have now, it might be hard to find someone who vomits, and she was right. I spent a whole day in the recovery room, and not one person vomited, although several were nauseous.

Once I was up on the wards, the nurses agreed to page me when someone was nauseous. I stayed at the hospital doing this volunteer work for 12 hours per day, for 14 days straight. My goal was to be able to stand beside the bed of someone vomiting or to hand them an emesis bowl. Even though I had gone through looking at pictures and videos (both movie scenes and a video of someone actually vomiting), I was still terrified of seeing it in real life. I was terrified enough that I didn't sleep very much, and woke up every morning for the first seven to ten days just dreading going back there.

My therapist asked me to call him every afternoon. After three or four days I called him crying, saying I didn't think I could continue. But I knew that this would mean I would never recover from the phobia because there was nothing left to work on in therapy. He responded with something I'll never forget. He said, "I believe in you." It was the most supportive thing anyone could have said in that moment, and it is something I say to many of my own patients when I know it to be true, which is more often than not.

Sure enough, only a day or two later I walked into a room and a patient was holding a little cardboard bowl under her chin. *This is it* I thought. *This is why I'm here.* I held my ground, and she vomited a tiny bit into the bowl. Well, you would have thought that I'd just won the 500-million-dollar lottery. After making sure my patient was alright I rushed to the locker room to telephone my therapist, my husband, and each of my three kids. I don't think any of them really understood my glee in that moment, but you probably will. I had already "conquered" the fear of eating, and then of being nauseous and vomiting years before. This was the final frontier.

The next few days in the hospital I was actually able to concentrate more on my job, and I found that I absolutely loved it! If I could have changed careers at that moment and become a hospital chaplain I would have. (Unfortunately, I would have needed to match with a hospital that needed chaplain residents and move across the country.)

Once I had finished celebrating, the next emotion I felt was extreme guilt about all the patients over the years who were members of my congregations whom I had neglected when they were in hospital. I either avoided them completely, or rushed in and rushed out, or stood there dissociated from reality, with no clue what they were telling me. In that short time in the hospital over those 14 days, I learned how rich of an experience it can be for people to just talk to someone about how they feel while they're in hospital. Some have life-changing or life-ending illnesses, and with me there as a volunteer, they got to reflect on the meaning of that for them. It was a service that the one overworked chaplain did not have time to give to every patient, and hospital budgets would never have room for more than one chaplain. So I decided to give back what I believe I had taken away with my negligence of people all those years. For the next five years I volunteered every Monday (my day off) at the hospital, picking up where I had left off. It was so wonderful I cannot describe it. When I walk into the hospital now and smell that familiar antiseptic smell, I get a warm, fuzzy feeling inside. It is the smell of my salvation.

If you don't have any friends or acquaintances in a local hospital, then perhaps ask your family doctor, minister, or priest to write a letter asking if you can spend some time there shadowing a nurse, social worker, or chaplain for a few days. You may also consider volunteering for the hospital auxiliary. These volunteers often deliver books and sundry items to patient rooms. They may also spend time with elderly patients who have no family to visit them. Nursing homes for the elderly and disabled are also a great place to do volunteer work.

REAL-LIFE EXPOSURES

1. Smell

You may have a fear of the smell of vomit, which is understandable because it smells like the depths of hell. By that I mean *nobody* likes it. Human beings are the only mammals with significant amounts of butyric acid in their digestive system. This acid is what gives vomit its obnoxious smell. Studies are currently being done on the benefit of taking more butyric acid as a supplement to help with irritable bowel syndrome (IBS) and other gut issues, so luckily, like everything else, it's for sale online. You can buy the acid in liquid form and mix up your own vomit recipe by adding it to a can of vegetable soup or stew. Do this experiment outside, as one of my patients did it inside and then texted me to ask how to get the smell out of her house. I didn't know the answer—sorry about that! If you don't have access to this acid you can do the same trick with Parmesan cheese, which is the only food that contains enough butyric acid to smell a bit like vomit.

2. Sight

Vomit looks terrible. I'm convinced that we perceive that so that we stay away from it. Other mammals don't seem to be bothered by what vomit looks like, but humans almost universally are grossed out. You've seen vomit by now in the pictures and videos you've watched, but you may wish to take it to the next step. It's easier if you get someone to help you do this by taking another can of soup or stew and throwing it somewhere that you get anxious about. That may be simply in the toilet, or you may need to do an exposure where you find it on the kitchen floor, or *almost* in the toilet. Seeing "vomit" in these places can help you to overcome the anxiety that rises up when you do. Remember, your goal is to *stay in the situation* and tolerate or accept the anxiety until it comes down on its own. Play the Raise Game as described in Chapter Two if at first it doesn't bother you.

3. Cleaning up

Most people with emetophobia don't seem to mind cleaning up vomit if they have children. I think I can safely say, I minded, but I did it because the only other alternative was dealing with the sick child, and I was thankful my husband was doing that. Some of my younger patients are so bothered by the sight of vomit, even animal vomit, that they can't clean it up. Still others are worried they won't know how to effectively clean vomit on carpeting or upholstery.

When I was a teenager, Mother and I had a cat who had kittens. Despite growing up on a farm, Mother didn't seem to know that all calico cats are female, and when a cat stomps its back feet rhythmically and meows loud and long, it's in heat. So we had kittens, but the deal was that I had to look after them and find homes for them. I readily agreed. I kept them in the basement on a soft rug that we put inside a black garbage bag. When they were old enough to eat something, and I can't remember what it was, they all vomited on this garbage bag, which was essentially their home. I cried when I saw it and ran upstairs. I told Mother I absolutely could not clean it up. Her response was this: "You go down there and clean that all up right now, or I will take every single one of those kittens and drown them." Yes, Mother was like that, and yes, she 100 percent would have done it. Nevertheless, it was probably a good thing. I sobbed and sobbed and cleaned up the vomit. After that, I was fine with cleaning up hairballs and whatnot, and eventually, I even began showing and breeding Persian cats in the early '80s, so there was a lot of ick to deal with. It probably helped me with raising my kids.

Cleaning up vomit on carpet or upholstery is easy enough if you have a steam cleaner. You can buy little portable ones for around $100 now, and they have a lot of benefits beyond vomit, such as detailing your car and really cleaning the furniture every once in a while. It almost costs as much to rent one as to buy one, and I've learned lately that most people with emetophobia don't want to rent them because they're afraid someone else rented it already to clean up vomit. I apologize if this thought never occurred to you, as it never did to me. So if you have a carpet cleaner you can purposely spill some soup on your carpet and practice cleaning it up. If you fear renting a carpet cleaner in general, then add this as one of your exposure exercises. Don't use any safety behaviors like bleaching it—just rent it and clean a carpet or a chair.

INSTRUCTIONS FOR CLEANING UP VOMIT

Begin by reading all these steps and ensuring you have everything you need. For example, you may wish to purchase the carpet cleaning solution in advance.

1. Pour a can of soup or stew on your carpet.
2. Don a mask and gloves.
3. Begin with taking a piece of cardboard and a dustpan to sweep up the majority of it. It's okay to throw the cardboard out, and you can clean the dustpan with a bleach solution later.
4. Once you only have stains to deal with, clean the carpet or upholstery with an electric carpet cleaner with the hottest water and a cleaning solution made specifically for vomit and feces (it will tell you on the bottle).
5. When you have finished, wash the plastic parts of the carpet cleaner in a bleach solution.
6. Throw away your mask and gloves and don't give it another thought. By this stage you should be far enough along with

your exposures to say to yourself, *It doesn't matter if I don't get every last particle of norovirus because if I catch it and I vomit, I can cope with it. I will be okay.*

4. Laundry

You may be afraid to do laundry that has been vomited on, such as pajamas or bed sheets. Virtually everything can be cleaned, so there is never a need to throw anything out. Try an exposure exercise around it by dumping another can of that soup or stew over someone's bed linen. It's okay to use gloves and a mask. You should shake out the majority of the fake vomit into your laundry sink. Then, wash the sheets and pajamas in hot water with bleach. Most hot water tanks and hot cycles on washing machines don't reach the 65°C needed to kill norovirus, so you need the bleach. Don't go crazy—½ cup per load will suffice.

5. Sounds

The sounds of vomiting that I listened to when I had emetophobia helped me incredibly, and they weren't as good as the ones I'm sharing with you here. I was particularly triggered by sound, and even if someone started coughing, I would run away or plug my ears, which was really embarrassing. Sounds were the worst for me at one time, although seeing someone vomit came to be worse in the end. It wasn't hard for me to figure out why. My dad was a loud vomiter, which is the understatement of the century. He made the weirdest sound when he was sick, and as he died of colon cancer, he was vomiting a lot in the end, which was awful for both of us. Dad made some sort of sound like "brrrrrr," over and over. I've never heard anyone else do this, even in a movie. I know that I'm not imagining it because his sister, my Aunt Murdena, told me she went to visit him in the hospital once and knew where his room was because she could hear him down the hall making that distinct sound.

Although I never found a sound like dad's, all the other sounds really got to me until I used them as an exposure exercise. Until the early 2000s I was afraid of ever being admitted to hospital *for any reason* or even going into the ER because they only draw a curtain between your beds, so you can hear everything. Once I did the exposure exercise with sounds I felt liberated from this fear! I no longer had to have anxiety about every little thing causing me a trip to the hospital. I could also stay upstairs and close to my family members in the house if they were sick, because hearing it no longer triggered me at all.

EXERCISE 1: Exposure—Listening to sounds

Listen to the three sound clips (via the QR code below), which are an amalgamation of various sounds. Some are not real, some are even funny (especially if you liked *The Walking Dead*), but most are real. I announce the title of the sound clip given by the person recording and submitting it, along with the number of seconds it takes. Try to listen to these sounds over and over until they simply don't bother you anymore, meaning your anxiety doesn't move from the baseline. Do the Raise Game (Chapter Two) if you're no longer bothered.

Once you can listen to these sounds you'll no longer need to plug your ears when you hear someone sick because the experience of listening to the ones I put together is far worse than anything you could hear in real life. Give yourself a big reward for getting through all the "virtual" exposures now, including those awful sounds. Go out to dinner with your beloved. If you can't afford dinner, make it a date night at home with a movie and a bottle of wine.

https://emetophobiahelp.org/figure-7-2/

EXERCISE 2: Establishing your avoidances

Write out all real-life things you avoid. Put them in order of easiest to do to most difficult. Integrate them into your safety behaviors calendar and begin working on them along with your other exposure homework.

EXERCISE 3: Exposure—Variability

It's now time to add "variability" to your lizard brain's learning experience. Researchers into exposure therapy have found that doing some easy and hard exposures with variety, as opposed to always in hierarchical order, can be beneficial.

Go to YouTube and type in "vomit," "puke," or "throw up," and watch whatever random videos show up. Some will be easy to see after the ones I selected for you in the previous chapter. Others may be shocking or more difficult. If they "haunt you" in the hours or days following, just like with pictures that are "burned" in your brain, the fix is to *go back and watch them again*. Avoiding them makes them much "bigger" in your brain to the point of catastrophic. Your adorable little assistance dog took you in the wrong direction, so redirect them *toward* what you fear!

SUMMARY

- I discussed how exposure exercises work if your main fear is yourself vomiting. Your brain generalizes learning, and tolerating higher anxiety levels (up to 6 or 7 on the SUD scale) over time trains the brain that is has been mistaken about vomiting being dangerous.
- Completing exposures also builds your confidence, so you are more likely to believe that you can cope with vomiting.
- Avoidance behaviors are harder to organize exposures around, but it is still possible. I discuss ways to end avoidance of things like driving, amusement parks, bars, schools, daycare, crowded places, family gatherings, and medical procedures. There may be a lot of planning involved, but the payoff is well worth it.
- I showed how to do real-life exposures to smell, sight, clean up, and sound.
- The final "virtual exposure" exercise is for "variability," by watching random vomit videos on YouTube. This step

is necessary to get used to something shocking you about vomiting. If a video "haunts" you, watch it again—avoidance only makes it worse.

Chapter Eight

LIVING WITH UNCERTAINTY

Life is uncertain, let's face it. It doesn't seem to matter anymore which part of the world you live in, there is an element of uncertainty. Climate change has brought torrential rain, blizzards, fires, and floods where there never were any before. People can lose their jobs at any time. In the cities, there are many temporary places to rent, but permanent rentals are disappearing such that regular folks are having to live in tents in the parks. Is anything for certain anymore?

I live along the Cascadia fault line that stretches north to us from California. The grandkids who live with us and attend school right behind our house have fire drills and earthquake drills. For an earthquake you have to get under your desk, so stuff doesn't fall on you. We've attached all our shelving to the walls, and we have an earthquake preparedness kit in our garden shed with enough food and water for a week, first aid supplies, and survival stuff. The big one that happened in Japan a few years ago really woke us up to the possibility, and since we live on an island at the mouth of the Fraser River as it empties into the ocean, we need to think about tsunamis as well. We're protected in part by Vancouver Island, but we can still get flooded right out of our house if it happens. So what do we do? Well, we prepare somewhat for the uncertainty, and then we just carry on with life and don't ever think about it. Although you're supposed to get under the kitchen table if there's an earthquake, we don't live under there. We go to work, we shop, we walk our dogs, and we sweep out our garages when all the stuff on the shelves out there could come crashing down and kill us at any moment over the next 50 years.

People with emetophobia need to understand that they must approach their lives in the sense of the uncertainty of vomiting in the same way that we here, on the West Coast, approach ours: never thinking of it. Can you imagine if I were paralyzed by an earthquake phobia? I would be sitting under the table right now with my laptop, trying to work. I'd rush out from under to get snacks and a glass of water, my heart beating at 150 bpm until I sank back under the table again to eat and drink. I might go get a pillow and blanket for the night, upset that I can't sleep in my own bed with my husband, or I would just lie awake, waiting for the shaking to start. Does all that seem crazy? I'm quite sure there are people just like that, just the same as there are people like you who may behave similarly about vomiting. It won't take much for you to make the comparison.

We risk life and limb every time we get into a car. In fact, your odds of dying in a car crash are about 1 percent, with similar odds of serious injury. Do you think about this every time you get behind the wheel? I doubt it—unless you also have a driving phobia. The fact is, you're just willing to risk something that could most certainly kill you. You send your kids to school, when they theoretically could get shot, and you go out shopping and to the movies, where *you* could theoretically get shot. I'm not trying to scare you, but it's still true that *we live with risk all the time*. So you need to do the same thing with vomiting. You need to risk it. There is no point in living under the kitchen table, right? So eat a hamburger without washing or sanitizing your hands first. That's what I'm talking about. Because unless you are willing to live with the risk that you might vomit, you'll never be fully recovered from the phobia.

Don't get me wrong: I wash my hands before I eat. But sometimes I can't, and that's okay. I just throw caution to the wind because that's good for me. Norovirus isn't the worst thing to happen to you. Emetophobia is.

CONTROL

We (you and I) would all love to be in control of everything even minutely related to vomiting all the time. It's probably got something to do with feeling so out of control as a child for a variety of reasons, none of which matters to your emetophobia recovery. Some psychologists have said that emetophobia is really about the need for control, although there is no evidence for this opinion. Emetophobia is about your lizard brain being triggered by things to do with vomiting, and consequently believing, at a deep-down level, that you'll die if you vomit. Never let anyone tell you that you're a "control freak." This is one of the most insensitive things anyone can say to someone who is phobic. Being called a control freak is one of those dismissive, thoughtless labels people throw around when they don't understand what's really going on. It's a lazy way to avoid seeing the bigger picture—that maybe you're someone who likes things orderly, who finds comfort in structure, or who's had to be in control because no one else would step up. It's not just rude; it's reductive, and it's often used to belittle someone's anxiety as if fear of chaos or unpredictability is something to mock. In truth, calling someone a control freak says more about the person saying it than the one being labelled.

Do we want to be in control? Of course, because *things* in our lives have always been out of control, and for sure we want to control vomiting as in stop it or avoid it all the live-long day. But we don't need to control everything in the world—only this.

Anyone with anxiety wants to control things related to their anxiety. My husband is always anxious about me digging holes in the yard in case we dig through a pipe of some kind. So he'd rather be the one doing the digging. He wants to control it because he's anxious about the outcome. You probably want to control things as well because you're anxious that if you don't, it could lead to someone catching a bug and passing it on to you. So some people with emetophobia control when their family members wash their hands, take showers, cook, and clean up. You probably always want to be in charge of cleaning if someone is sick because you don't trust anyone else to isolate that person or clean up as well as you. This can lead to that age-old insult: "control freak."

All the same, you *do* need to let go of control of all these situations. They're safety behaviors at best, and at worst they're behaviors that keep you continuing to believe that vomiting is something catastrophic and awful like a war or a natural disaster that has to be avoided at all costs. It isn't, it's just vomiting. Just a bodily function to help you out if you're sick or poisoned. So you don't need to control other people or situations that may be about germs, contamination, or other things that lead to vomiting.

THE INFORMATION AGE

I think the internet, including social media, is to blame for a lot of the behavior people with emetophobia have today. As my phobia existed and was successfully treated before the internet, I didn't know about norovirus or other germs, food poisoning, or any other situations like overexertion in exercise, or migraine headaches, or childbirth, all of which the internet tells me can lead to vomiting. So I feel for you, reading this book, in this "Information Age," which could also aptly be called the "Misinformation Age." No matter what information you have learned on social media or by Googling things, the treatment for your phobia is the same: slowly expose yourself to what you fear, stop avoiding, and give up safety behaviors. Some people on a journey to end their emetophobia actually give up their social media until they believe they are recovered from the phobia. I understand that this is difficult to do because I, too, at 66 years of age, am addicted to TikTok and Instagram. To keep up with the lives of my other senior citizen friends I need to stay on Facebook. To laugh out loud every day I have to stick with X. I feel for you, Millennials, Generation Z, and now, my littlest grandkids tell me, Generation Alpha. (I guess we're starting the alphabet designations again at the beginning.)

Living in the Information Age with social media is a good exposure, however, in living with uncertainty. We have no idea when we're going to see someone vomiting on TikTok. Or when a moms' group on Facebook is going to go on and on about how bad norovirus is this year. Our cousin will even post a picture of her sick kid on Instagram with a bowl beside his bed, and we have no control over that. It's okay. Lean into it. We have spent so much of our lives avoiding what we fear that even with the mild triggers we "lean away," meaning we do things like scroll quickly past. *Leaning in* means that you will actually stop scrolling or watch the video two or three times just to make sure you're no longer avoiding it. Lean in to any and all activities that might result in you catching norovirus because it's a harmless virus that's over in a day or two.

MY NOROVIRUS STORY

Even after all the work I did over 25 long years to overcome emetophobia, there was still one last obstacle I had yet to overcome: norovirus.

It probably took me 25 years, for one reason because it's not like I'm going to sign up for norovirus just to prove a point to myself. Although I was still leading a fairly hygienic lifestyle, I wasn't thinking about vomiting all day every day anymore, so it was easy for my mind to slip. This happened when I moved my daughter from Vancouver to a city called Edmonton, which is in the northern part of the next province of Alberta. The drive is about 12 or 13 hours if you don't stop. We decided we needed to take two cars since she had a fair amount of stuff and a giant German Shepherd in a crate. So my daughter and I and the dog set out in one car and her husband and mine in the other. The menfolk were going to drive back after leaving my daughter's car and I was going to fly back about a week later.

En route, we stopped for gas and bought a container of loose candy like gummy bears and such. I pumped the gas and my daughter took over the driving. As she was the only one to go inside, I didn't think to wash my hands after pumping the gas (I know, I know). I handed her candy out of the bag, and I ate the candy as well. We got her moved in, and the next night, we all ate a nice dinner together before the men left to return home. Just about exactly 24 hours after we had arrived, I said that instead of going out for a walk with Liz and the dog, I would stay in, as I really wasn't feeling well. I took some Gravol® because the nausea was getting worse. Right after Liz left with the dog, at about 9 pm, I started with the explosions out the back end, and within an hour, I was also vomiting. Liz began to not feel well after the dog walk and started vomiting at about 11 pm. We knew it wasn't food poisoning because the men had eaten what we had eaten and they were fine. I also had come to the realization of what I had done with not washing my hands at the gas station about 24 hours earlier.

Our predicament was kind of funny, in hindsight. We were in a basement apartment, and the landlady was upstairs, although she could easily come down the stairs and would arrive right in the living room, something she had to do to get to the laundry room. Other than briefly meeting the landlady, we didn't know a soul in Edmonton. And, of course, there was only one washroom in the basement suite. For the life of me, I don't know how we managed not to have to use that washroom at the same time, but we did. We really didn't want to have to go upstairs and beg to throw up in the landlady's washroom. At one point, when I was in the washroom, my daughter used a bucket, but she stood right outside the washroom door, so I could hear her vomiting. We laugh about that a lot now. To be honest, it wasn't the vomiting that worried either of us—it was having to sit on the toilet because no one wants to have to use a bucket instead of a toilet in their own house.

We were sick off and on throughout that night, but felt better in the morning. The worst part for me was not being able to keep down my medication for chronic pain, so I was suffering pretty badly. I was also "taking notes" to help my various patients and people online who ask me questions. For example, I had a stopwatch and learned that it only takes 3 seconds to vomit. Three measly seconds and yet a whole lifetime of being afraid of it!

The next morning we were sitting at the kitchen table sipping apple juice and staring into oblivion. My daughter suddenly said, "Mum, you weren't scared at all."

"Oh yeah," I replied. "Huh."

I didn't even think about being scared. Yes, I took the Gravol®, but that was because the nausea was really bad and painful, and I thought it might just go away. But once I started vomiting I just thought, *Oh man, here we go, I've caught something.* Fear didn't even enter into any part of my reality. And afterward, when I thought about it, I can promise you it was not nearly as bad as I'd imagined it would be. Not even one one-millionth as bad. Yes, I vomited a few times over the course of the night, but after you've done it once, the rest of the times don't seem to matter.

I know that some people with emetophobia get norovirus and experience it in a different way. Sometimes they're so scared it makes their phobia worse. But I honestly think that the worst part, for all of them, is the way they feel about it and not what is actually happening. By that I mean the worst part is the anxiety. You see, I don't think that you are truly afraid of vomiting. You are afraid of the terrifying, horrific, out-of-control panic you're going to feel right before. It's the panic that is intolerable and not the vomiting. Hence, your problem is not vomiting; it's anxiety. Your anxiety is out of control, and you need to work on that—you don't need to waste one more second of your life thinking about vomiting because it is 100 percent not the problem you have.

ARE YOU LEANING IN?

Our emetophobia can be so subtle we don't even notice it sometimes. I remember about 10 years ago, long after I was fully recovered, we were arranging cars to drive 45 minutes back from my daughter's bakery to our home. Originally I was supposed to ride in the middle back seat between two other people. I did not have any expectation that one of them would vomit as everyone seemed healthy and happy. But I just said, "I'll wait for Charlie," which would mean riding in the front seat with only my husband. This was subtle avoidance. It was leaning away, rather than into, the phobia. And I could have kicked myself later for doing it. It was one of those times when I really had to sit and think about how I could have behaved differently, what would be the warning signs that I was about to avoid or lean away, etc. The next time something like this came up, where I had to sit in the back of the car between two kids in car seats, I did it! And, of course, it was fine. I even told myself that if one of them was sick I'd be okay, it wouldn't be a big deal. So I encourage you to think long and hard about what kinds of things you need to lean into rather than away from. Make a list. Lean in.

The force of avoidance in our lizard brains is like a strong current in a river. I remember a time when I was out hiking with my dog, a German Shepherd who loved the water (see Figure 8.1). The Fraser River is wide and deep, and the current is incredibly strong. My dog ran off, way upriver, and then decided to jump into the water, but the current quickly carried her to a nearby shore around the bend of the river where she couldn't see me. I thought I was a strong swimmer at the time, and the river looked completely calm, so I jumped in, to swim upstream to her, about 100 feet. I swear it took me an hour like I was in one of those special pools they make just so you can work out but not get anywhere. I felt like the dog was cheering me on, somehow, and I finally got to where she was, grabbed her collar, and the two of us swam back to where I started in under a minute, being carried gleefully by the invisible current. When I was swimming upstream *against* the current I was almost overwhelmed with how much energy, effort and work it was going to take my little 120-pound body (at the time) to get to where I was going. I almost gave up, but I needed to get to my dog. Afterwards, I was reflecting on the experience and thought that it was just about the same as my work in overcoming emetophobia. Swimming upstream against a strong current. Oh how easy it would be to just turn around and go back! But in the river and with my emetophobia work I felt the same: I could not give up, despite the strong force pushing me in the opposite direction to where I wanted to go.

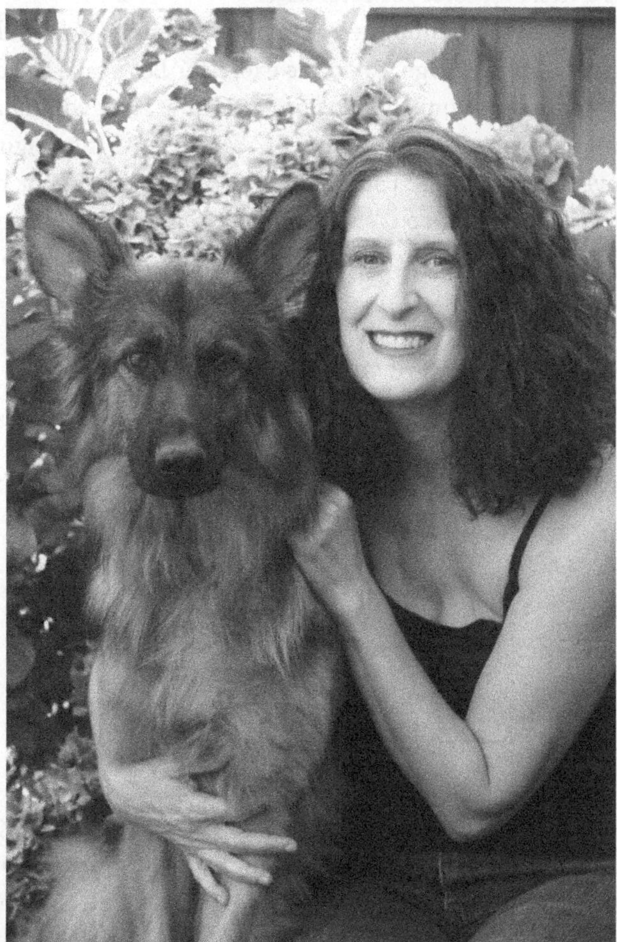

Figure 8.1. Anna and Guinness

COURAGE AND WILLINGNESS

About this time you may be thinking *Anna, I'm not ready to do all the things you're suggesting.* I get that. I also get that you're probably more ready than you think you are—it's just a lot of work to do them. So, given the strength of the force of avoidance, how are you ever going to do the exercises in this book and finally conquer this phobia once and for all? I suggest that being able to do any given task is based on both willingness and courage. How courageous do you believe you are, in general, from 1–100, with 100 being the most courageous? Figure 8.2 shows a thermometer for reference.

The other factor is willingness. The test is simple: how willing are you, in terms of percentage, to do the exercise? Let's take the exercise of watching random vomit videos on YouTube. How willing are you to do it? 50 percent willing? 10 percent? 80 percent? (See Figure 8.3.)

I believe that courage is something you're born with or develop very early in childhood, so it's not really possible to get more. But it is always possible to become more willing to do something, no matter how courageous you feel.

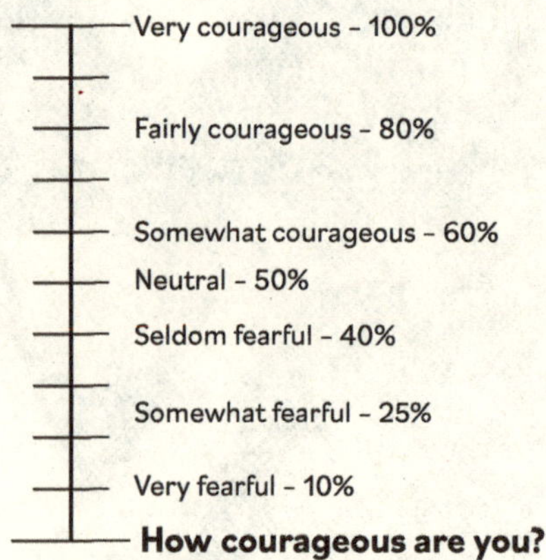

Figure 8.2. Levels of courage

I firmly believe that any percentage number that you've recorded at 50 percent or above means that you're willing to do it. You might be thinking, *but I'm only halfway there*. No, your willingness is halfway there but your courage may be all the way there. That is to say, *I believe in you*. I have been encouraging my emetophobic patients for over a decade now and I don't think I've been wrong in this regard. Sure, some of them refuse to do the exercise, but that doesn't mean they couldn't have managed it.

Exposure exercise	**Willingness (%)**
Watching these videos (list below):	
Listening to these sounds:	
Giving up these safety behaviors:	
Smelling vomit (butyric acid, BARFume, Parmesan cheese)	
Cleaning up fake vomit	
Getting near toilets	
Pretend-vomiting these things:	
Supporting a person fake vomiting	
Experiencing exercise-induced nausea	
Experiencing dizziness	
Eating vomit-flavored jellybeans	
Gagging yourself	

Figure 8.3. Exposures and willingness

I would measure my courage level at below average—perhaps about 30 or 40. You may think, given my life story, that I would measure much higher, but I am, in fact, a big chicken. I spent most of my young life doing ballet and now I play curling with a helmet on. Not exactly life-threatening stuff. I loved gymnastics as a kid but was too afraid of the bars and the vault to continue. I'm afraid of people being angry, yelling at me, or not liking me. I'm afraid of answering my phone because it could be someone calling with the intent to do what's in the aforementioned sentence. I'm afraid of anything new or doing anything under a time pressure. I have an extremely low pain threshold. How did such a woosy-woos like me ever recover from emetophobia? Well, because willingness I have in spades (see Figure 8.4).

THE WILLINGNESS/COURAGE QUADRANTS

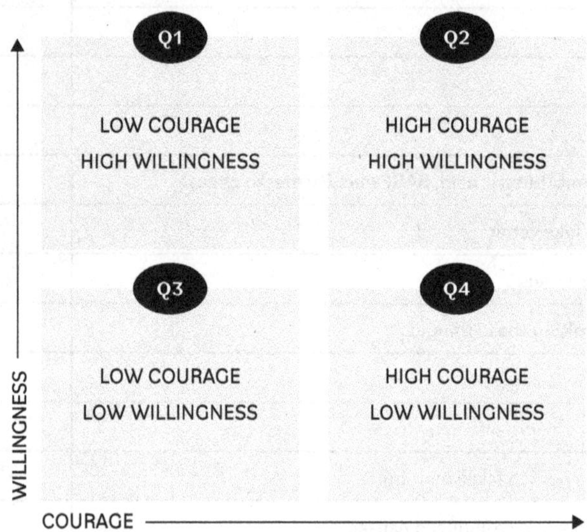

Figure 8.4. Willingness/courage quadrants

1. Quadrant 1: Low courage, high willingness. This is where I reside. I was willing to do whatever it took to get over the phobia, but I was terrified doing it all the time. High willingness could be indicative of your intellectual ability to use reason and logic to help train your brain.

2. Quadrant 2: High courage, high willingness. Lucky you! It may be difficult to get maximum benefit from exposures because they don't raise your anxiety enough. Playing the Raise Game (Chapter Two) will be necessary at most levels.

3. Quadrant 3: Low courage, low willingness. This is the most difficult quadrant to reside in. You may be depressed, and once your depression is treated you will find that both courage and willingness levels rise enough to do the exercises. You may need more optimism and hope and thus encouragement from support persons or reading stories of others who have gone through the exposures and beaten the odds.

4. Quadrant 4: High courage, low willingness. You're probably a person who can easily cope with the feelings you'll experience while doing the exposures and exercises in this book. However, you may tend to procrastinate. You'll need support and accountability to start it and stick with it.

If you're stalling on doing the exercises and exposures, ask yourself what obstacles are still lying in your way. You can't become more courageous, as that is basically innate, but you can certainly become more willing. If you have been diligently working through the exercises in this book, one after the other, then you should, by now, have run into at least one thing that was hard to do, perhaps you may have found it impossible even, but you did it and surprised yourself. Some task lay in your path all along that you managed to bowl over and complete. How did you do it? Did you muster up courage that you never thought you had? Did your support person offer you encouragement? Did you finally get fed up with yourself avoiding it all the time?

I remember when I was working on pictures of people vomiting. I was too afraid to look at one of them, as it was described, so I had my husband click on the link to it, print it out, and put it in a file folder so I could take it to my next therapy appointment. I figured my therapist would have some sort of magical way to help me open the file. The file folder sat on our dining room table for about three days until I finally said to myself *Oh for God's sake* and just opened it. The picture was nasty, and I got a bit of a shock, but it's not like anything bad happened to me. You may have had a similar experience with certain exercises in this book. Sometimes becoming more willing is like finding our *Oh for God's sake* moment.

You can apply the willingness/courage test to many things in your life, not just this phobia. Whenever you find yourself afraid to do something or try something, do the willingness/courage test. How willing are you to cut out sugar from your diet? To start going to the gym? How about to paint the outside of your house yourself?

You may find that you are willing to do an exercise, but can't seem to muster up the courage.

EXERCISE 1: Reviewing safety behaviors

Review your safety behaviors calendar and check how you're doing.

List any obstacles you think may be holding you back from giving these behaviors up.

Add all your avoidance behavior exposure exercises to your calendar.

Include watching random videos on your calendar.

If you feel you can't complete any of these exposure exercises, write down what you believe may be holding you back and then do the willingness/courage test for each exercise. There are more exposures to come in Chapters Nine and Ten!

SUMMARY

- Life is full of uncertainty, from climate disasters to car accidents, yet we don't live in constant fear of them. You must learn to live with uncertainty and lean into the things that trigger you.
- Avoiding vomiting at all costs is like hiding under a table all day for fear of an earthquake—it's no way to live. Take small risks, like eating without washing your hands every time.
- The idea that emetophobia is about control is misleading. You're not a "control freak." It's about the brain's deep-seated

belief that vomiting is a life-threatening event. Nevertheless, you must still give up control of everything about germs and vomiting.

- The internet makes emetophobia worse by bombarding people with information about norovirus, food poisoning, and other potential vomiting triggers. Leaning into triggers rather than avoiding them is key.
- Avoidance can be so ingrained it happens automatically.
- Facing fears is like swimming against a strong current.
- The willingness/courage test helps you see why you may not be able to do the work, and what to do to overcome this.
- Sometimes, overcoming fear is about reaching an *Oh for God's sake* moment—getting so fed up with yourself that you just do it.

Chapter Nine

INTEROCEPTIVE WORK

Interoception is the awareness of internal bodily sensations, such as heart rate, breathing, hunger, fullness, temperature, pain, and emotional feelings. Since so many people with emetophobia fear their own bodies, interoceptive work is important in working to overcome it. Although people with emetophobia are notoriously bad at interoception, meaning that we *mis*interpret bodily sensations all the time, I think Mother explaining a lot of my bodily sensations to me when I was a child helped me. That, and the fact that there was no internet to contradict her. Perhaps it was just my personality type, or that I wanted to believe her, and so I did. As I've said before, taking part in an ERP group where we recorded our amount of anxiety and our amount of nausea after each exposure showed me that the two were linked.

Despite the way I overcame the interoceptive part of emetophobia, I quickly came to realize when working with patients that no amount of explaining their symptoms or writing down nausea levels seemed to help them much. I learned about interoceptive exposures when I did my CBT and OCD training, and I began collecting ideas for people with emetophobia at that time.

Interoceptive exercises are those that help the patient become more aware of bodily sensations. It can be as simple as stopping to be mindful of how your body feels: are your shoulders stiff? Are your legs tense? How are you breathing right now? Take a moment to analyze how your body feels at this very moment and try not to include anything to do with stomach or intestinal discomfort. I've given you some examples in the following chart (Figure 9.1).

Headache?	☐
Allergies/sinus issues?	☐
Sore/stiff neck?	☐
Tight shoulders?	☐
Tight arms and wrists?	☐
Sweaty hands/fingers curled?	☐
Sore back?	☐
Tight hips?	☐
Tight legs?	☐
Tight knees?	☐
Tight feet/toes curled?	☐
I feel pretty good!	☐
I need coffee.	☐

Figure 9.1. Body feelings chart

EXERCISE 1: Morning awareness

As a person with emetophobia, you are probably paying way too much attention to your body, especially your stomach and related areas. It may be the first thing you notice when you wake up in the morning. Tomorrow morning, see if you can notice the first thing you *hear* when you wake up. Keep doing this until it becomes second nature to listen for sounds rather than scanning your body for signs of illness.

These exercises, like everything else in your recovery journey, may have to be done for many months before they become entirely effective.

EXERCISE 2: Keeping a symptoms journal

I advise all my patients who pay too much attention to their bodies to keep a symptoms journal for one month. This exercise is important, not for the results, but for the *way* the journal is kept. Here is an example of a symptoms journal:

Month:

Day	Symptoms description	Did I vomit?

Figure 9.2. Symptoms journal

Write down your symptom (the way your stomach/body feels) every time you feel a sensation that makes you afraid or worry. Come back to the journal 24 hours later and write "Yes" or "No" in the column "Did I vomit?"

Now you and I both know, before you even start, that you're going to write "No" every single time. But that doesn't matter. As I said, it's not the result we're looking for; it's the *process* of keeping the journal. Coming back, day after day, for a month or more, and writing "No" will slowly train that lizard brain that these symptoms are not worth focusing on. Once you've written in your symptoms, try not to actively think about them again. By actively, I mean reassuring yourself, entering into a discussion or arguing with the thoughts, or calling your anxiety a monster.

It is important for you to do interoceptive exposure exercises now as part of your ERP work. The purpose of the exercises is not to vomit, as that is not necessary, but rather, it is to do something you would normally avoid because you fear it might make you vomit, and to get used to noticing those feelings in your body but leaving them alone instead of focusing on them. Again, you have to throw caution to the wind a bit here. If you've been conscientiously doing all the exercises in this book as you go along, you should be at the point now where you are able to think, *It doesn't matter if I vomit anyway because I know it won't hurt me*. So interoceptive exercises are meant to make you feel sick. You're ready for it!

EXPOSURE: INTEROCEPTIVE WORK

EXERCISE 3: Dizziness

You are likely afraid of getting dizzy because you know that some people vomit when they're dizzy even if you never have. So it's time to make yourself feel dizzy. This is easy to do because all you have to do is stand in the center of a room and spin around. Keep spinning long after you feel the dizziness. When you're good and dizzy sit down and let yourself experience how it feels. Remind yourself that it's okay if you vomit—it won't be a big deal, and it will prove to you once and for all that you can vomit and nothing bad will happen. Put a garbage can with a liner nearby, just to make sure. This will also serve as an added exposure.

EXERCISE 4: Toilet exposure

Many people with emetophobia I have met and talked to online have a fear of toilets related to their emetophobia. By fear, I mean they are often disgusted by being around a toilet and/or they're afraid to vomit into one for a variety of reasons. Many people with emetophobia say they'd rather vomit outside, or into a garbage bag that they then throw away. This is understandable, as the very sight of toilets triggers their emetophobia anxiety. By now, you will understand what we do with triggers: exposure exercises! Practice coming into the washroom, lifting up the seat of the toilet, and kneeling down in front of it. Use the STAR plan, as described in Chapter Two.

You may need to retreat from your place at the toilet if your anxiety is too high to tolerate and none of the calming actions work for you this time. If you can't lift the seat of the toilet at first, just kneel down. If you can't kneel, then stand. Keep working at this exposure until you're comfortable with being around the toilet, and then you are ready for the following interoceptive exercise.

EXERCISE 5: Pretend-vomiting

Pretending to vomit can be quite scary, probably because a lot of people with emetophobia believe it might cause it to happen. If you feel that way, it's a good exposure to do! Start by filling your mouth with water. Lean over the toilet and spit it out while making some kind of nasty vomiting sound. You can do this when no one is around so you're not embarrassed, or you can have someone with you at first, if you think it might be easier.

Once you've mastered pretend-vomiting the water, graduate to a mouthful of breakfast cereal or oatmeal, and spit that into the toilet. It will look bad once it's in the toilet, adding another dimension to your exposure exercise. Practice flushing it away. Practice not quite making it all into the toilet and cleaning it up yourself.

The next thing to try pretend-vomiting is another can of that soup or stew. Nobody likes putting cold condensed soup or stew into their mouth—yetch!—so it will be a great exposure exercise. Remember leaning in? Swimming upstream? You can do it! I had one patient, a therapist herself, who stirred up ham, scalloped potatoes, and mixed carrots and peas to practice vomiting with because that was what she ate the last time she vomited. That was very brave on her part. Think about whatever might make you actually feel sick and use that.

EXERCISE 6: Fake-vomiting in public

Now perhaps you're ready to try pretend-vomiting in a public toilet. This exercise can be very effective for those of you who have social anxiety or fear of embarrassment from vomiting in public. You can start by just going into a cubicle when no one else is in the public washroom, and when you hear someone enter, start some fake vomiting sounds. You don't need to spit anything into the toilet, although if you take a water bottle in with you, you can certainly try that. Do this exercise a number of times and see how people react when you come out of the cubicle. You may find that many people ask if you're alright. Some others may be disgusted or stay away from you in case you're contagious. Neither of these responses is dangerous to you and need not be feared. Embarrassment is uncomfortable, but you can tolerate it, particularly if you practice.

If you feel really brave you can take a big sip of water, wander around a mall or public place for a while (such as a crowd at a concert or even a parade), and then fake-vomit the water into a garbage can in public. If you do this, you can see the reaction of a lot of people. Remember that although you may know intellectually what the reaction of others will probably be, your lizard brain does not know until you *experience* it.

EXERCISE 7: Support person "vomiting"
It can be a really helpful exposure exercise to have your significant other pretend to vomit in the toilet while you stand there beside them. If you have kids and your goal is ultimately to be close to them while they vomit, then practice this exposure until you can sit on the floor next to them and rub their back or just touch them. I have found that most spouses are totally down for this exposure exercise, and will probably find it humorous. You can go a step further if you dare and have them fake-vomit the vegetable soup but miss the toilet bowl and get it everywhere. Then you need to clean it up. This can be a challenge, but it's probably best to try doing this when at least there is no vomit smell.

EXERCISE 8: Exercise-induced nausea
Check with your doctor before trying this exercise. If you are particularly fit and workout in a gym or are on a sports team, then this exercise may not work for you. But if you're like most people in the Western world, you're somewhere between walk-the-dog-daily and couch potato. Beginning an exercise program, particularly if you decide to work until near exhaustion, will cause your muscles to release lactic acid. This acid is produced when breaking down glucose and converting it to energy. If you have a high energy demand, your muscles will not only produce lactic acid, but also will release toxins that may have been stored in them. This excess of lactic acid and toxins makes people feel nauseous, and some may even vomit. The vomiting may also be due to a reduction of blood flow to the digestive system, stalling it and making you feel sick as a result.

The exercise, if allowed by your doctor, will be to do a cardio workout until you feel exhausted. This workout can be as simple as jumping jacks in your living room or running on the spot. You can also run on a treadmill if you have one, or dust off any exercise machines you have stored at the back of your closet.

Once you've worked out until exhaustion, sit down and notice how you feel. Allow the nausea to be there and don't do anything to try to reduce or stop it. Resist all temptation to use a safety behavior. Allow yourself to feel terrible, knowing that the feeling will not hurt you, even if it does make you vomit. Nothing about this feeling is at all dangerous, so you need not fear it.

Once you've done this exercise and felt your anxiety come down, be sure to drink a sports drink or at the very least enough water to rehydrate you. Sports drinks will replace the sugar, salt, and electrolytes in your body, and will help a lot with muscle recovery.

EXERCISE 9: Jellybean exposure

If you're a fan of the Harry Potter series of books by J.K. Rowling, you'll remember that the Weasley twins sold packs of every flavor of jellybean, including vomit-flavored. Apparently, these are sold in stores and online you can find them quite easily. There is also a game called Beanboozled, which has participants spinning a wheel that lands on a color. You have to eat the jellybean of that color, and each color has a nice flavor and a horrid one, so you never know what you might get.

I bought this game just to try it out. We set up the game around the table and I gave everyone a compost bag to put in front of them in case they had to spit out a bean or in case they vomited. My grandson, aged eight at the time, said with enthusiasm and a huge grin, "I hope I throw up!" No one vomited while playing the game, but I can tell you from experience that the worst flavor was not vomit—it was a tie between canned dog food and dirty dishwater.

Beanboozled is a great game to play for an exposure exercise, even if you play it alone, as not knowing what flavor you might get adds *variability* to your exposures. Once you have advanced to the interoceptive stage of your exposure work, you should be ready to mix things up a bit. Not knowing if your jellybean might taste like peach or like vomit is a great way to do this. The idea is that life is not predictable. Things get thrown at us left and right all the time, and we need to be either prepared for it or learn how to go with the flow.

EXERCISE 10: Practice gagging

Gagging is something that most people with emetophobia really fear. It's normal to gag when you vomit as the vomit comes up past your gag reflex. Gagging brings something from the back of your throat into your mouth and prevents you from swallowing it. But because of its close association with vomiting, and even retching or dry heaving, gagging has become a huge trigger for people with emetophobia. I, myself, had to learn that gagging didn't mean I would vomit, and I learned this exactly in the way I'm about to describe.

Take a popsicle stick, the handle of a spoon, or your toothbrush, and move it to the back of your tongue until you gag. This is best done at the sink in front of a mirror. You may need to try this in stages if you're very frightened of it. Once you've tried it a few times to get used to the gagging feeling, try doing it in a public washroom or a public place!

Some of the aforementioned smells may make you gag in and of themselves. Try smelling something foul while gagging yourself. If you vomit, so what? It won't hurt you. Try to remember that it doesn't matter if you vomit—not during these exercises—not ever.

EXERCISE 11: Fun reward

Playing a fun game with your family is a great reward after these difficult exercises and I think, after I've now suggested two games (the Raise Game (Chapter Two) and Beanboozled) that were not the least bit fun, that I owe you one. Our family (with three kids) loved a game called Six. Set up a cap, a scarf, two oven mitts, a knife and fork, and a big, delicious chocolate bar on a table. On another table, the family rolls one die. When someone rolls a six everyone yells "Six!" and the person who rolled it runs around the other table twice, then dons the cap, scarf and oven mitts, and proceeds to eat the chocolate bar with a knife and fork. However, the rest of the family keeps rolling the dice, so if another person rolls a six, the first person must stop what they're doing and return to the family table. This game involves the sharing of utensils, so it's a good exposure for you when played within a family.

EXERCISE 12: Deepened extinction

Yes, I'm sorry to tell you, there's more. Just when you thought you'd mastered everything! Deepened extinction helps you even more to eliminate the fear from your lizard brain and your body. To put it simply, deepened extinction is just doing two exposure exercises (preferably one being interoceptive) at the same time. So you can put on one of the sound clips, perhaps in your earbuds, and try spinning around until you're very dizzy. There are a plethora of possibilities. Smell the BARFume or Parmesan cheese and watch a vomiting video at the same time. The chart in Figure 9.3 will help you to set up and practice some deepened extinction exercises.

But wait, there's more!

Begin by finding the number "1." It will be located in a square on a row that leads horizontally to "When not feeling well" and vertically to "Eat a big meal." This is your exposure exercise. A "big meal" may be simply eating at a time when you wouldn't want to eat (as a safety behavior), or it could mean taking one or two bites more after you're full. Did you have dessert? Unless you're obese, diabetic, or have stopped eating sugar, then for goodness sake, have dessert. Enjoy it.

After completing exercise "1" search for the "2," and so on. There are 34 exposure exercises in total. Once you've completed all 34, go back and start again. And again. Until none of these things gives you any anxiety.

	Eat a big meal	Listen to sounds	Watch a vomit video	Smell vomit mixture	Fake vomiting	Spin around	Taste vomit beans	Gag yourself
After eating a big meal			14				30	31
When not feeling well	1	8	15	21	26	28	31	32
While listening to sounds	2							
While watching a vomit video	3							
While smelling vomit mixture	4	9	16					
While fake vomiting in a toilet	5	10	17	22				
While spinning around	6	11	18	23				After spinning – 33
While tasting vomit beans	7	12	19	24	27	29		After tasting – 34
While gagging yourself	13	20	25					

Figure 9.3. Deepened extinction chart

EXERCISE 13: Further deepened extinction

Further deepened extinction is simply doing exposure exercises in groups of three or more. I've found that with people with emetophobia, one of these two things is easy to use as a starting point: eating a big meal, or eating much more than you would normally; and not feeling well (doing exercises on a day or at a time when you're already nauseous).

- Eat a big meal, listen to sounds, and pretend to vomit into a toilet.
- Start out on a day when you don't feel well, put on a vomiting video, and gag yourself.
- Eat more than normal, go out in public, and listen to sounds with your earbuds.
- You can use your imagination, or work from the chart in Figure 9.3.

EXERCISE 14: Make a plan

I've managed to pack a lot of exercises and ideas into this chapter. So that you're not overwhelmed it's probably best to make a plan. You can use another blank calendar or write out your plan in a journal or notebook. What exposures are you planning to do each day? Have you been working away at them as you've been reading this book or are you behind or not even started yet? I suggest working through at least all the exposures on our emetophobia.net website along with making a calendar, and finally, writing out a plan. Remember that you must give up all of your safety behaviors, which includes things you avoid. You'll know that you've succeeded in beating this phobia when you can say to yourself, *It doesn't matter if I vomit* and mean it.

SUMMARY

- Interoceptive work is crucial as a final step to overcoming emetophobia.
- You likely misinterpret body sensations, overfocusing on stomach feelings while ignoring everything else. Exercises help retrain your brain to tolerate normal bodily discomforts.
- Deepened extinction, or combining two exercises, makes exposure even more effective.
- Further deepened extinction, or combining three or more exposures, pushes you even harder.
- You made a plan for the final stages of recovery.

Chapter Ten

LIVING YOUR LIFE

I find it hard to put into words what it's like to live my life without emetophobia. My journey took 25 years, but it need not have. If anyone had been familiar with treatment for emetophobia when I was a child, if there had been a book like this one or resources such as those I offer now for therapists, it may have only taken me a year or two to recover. My life may have taken me in a completely different direction if there had been research, publications, books, or an internet, but I don't regret this long journey. It has ultimately led me to the most fulfilling and exciting career at the end of my working life. There is nothing better on this earth than getting an email from someone who had emetophobia, thanking me for my podcast, my book for therapists, my classes, my individual help, or one of my websites. Every time a person with emetophobia can meet a goal, such as caring for their child or travelling to see a loved one, it warms my heart.

Recovery from emetophobia is still a long road, as compared to having a phobia of puppies, for example. We can get someone over a dog phobia in two hours. And guess what? At the end of their treatment, those people get a puppy. What do we get? You guessed it: vomit. But it is satisfying and wonderful at the same time to sit with a sick child or go on a trip with family or even eat out at a restaurant with your significant other when you never have before. I hope this book will take you to those places, but do not expect to get there quickly. Most people I work with have to work diligently for one to two years to completely eradicate the phobia of vomiting from their life. I'd say the majority of people I see still have trouble doing that. They go so far—perhaps through all the exposure exercises I have online—and then they stall. That's because continued work is hard, and it's not nearly so structured and straightforward. That ladder gets scary near the top. By the end, you may feel as if you've slipped down a rung or two or had to reach for a rung by standing on your tiptoes, risking a slip or fall. You may hold on by your fingertips, hoping, praying, until you can catch the rung with the other hand and climb up. It feels great, though! Or it should. Be sure you're giving yourself enough credit for the difficult work you're doing when you finally accomplish each goal.

I now live in a big house in a suburb of Vancouver with one of my daughters, her husband, and their two children, who are, at this writing, 12 and 9 years old. We have all lived together for about 14 years now. It's been like a reset or a second chance for me. While I ran away from my own kids when they were sick, freaked out, and broke down into inconsolable tears, now I can look after my grandkids when they're sick. A while ago I volunteered to sit in the washroom with my granddaughter who had been vomiting all night as her parents were exhausted. I've taken kids in the car as well and had one of them be sick and it was fine. I've flown to Germany and all over Canada many times, gone to the dentist, and booked medical appointments, with no anxiety about them.

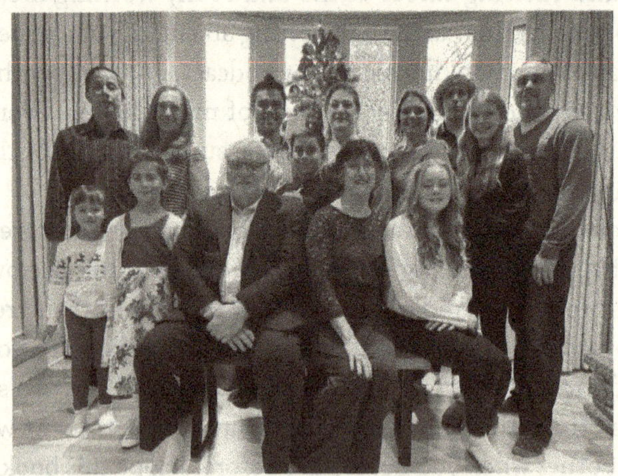

Figure 10.1. My whole family

I have a big family now. Holidays can be a logistical nightmare, but both my son and middle daughter have houses big enough for all of us (see Figure 10.1). If my sister comes along with her daughter, two grandkids, and now a great grandson (age three), the 20 of us are a wild zoo of entertainment and joy. Most of our major holidays (and birthdays) are in the winter when it's cold and flu season, so someone is always getting sick or getting over being sick. Until writing this, I don't think I've ever thought of that. Just imagine that, for a moment.

IT'S NEVER PERFECT

Once I had breast cancer I was told to have yearly mammograms, and they always made me anxious. No longer having emetophobia, I had something new to be worried about. As I was scheduled for my mammogram every October, I would start worrying about it around the end of August, which is ridiculous. Often the mammogram would show something weird, and I'd have to go to the Women's Hospital in Vancouver for a follow-up with a better machine. They'd decide it was nothing and I'd be done for another year. My doctor told me in my 40s I'd be dealing with this for the next 40 years. The other option was to have a double mastectomy reconstruction, without implants, but using fat from my abdomen to make new breasts. This operation would take about 10 hours. Without emetophobia to worry about I readily agreed and had the surgery in 2009. It ended up taking 14 hours and let me tell you, I felt like a barn floor when I woke up from that. Sure enough, the first thing I said was "I'm afraid I'm going to be sick." They put a little cardboard dish next to me and told me to turn my head. They didn't get that I had no intention of vomiting—I was just afraid. But there it was again, that old phobia just sneaking back in when my wits weren't about me.

To make matters worse, I had to be wheeled into a super-hot room for 24 hours so that my blood vessels would dilate because blood flow to the new breasts was important to keep them alive. A nurse came into my room once an hour for 24 hours and listened with a Doppler ultrasound to hear that blood was still flowing through them. So I was hot, irritated, sleep-deprived, and nauseous beyond all belief. Every four hours they hung an IV bag of Gravol®. I'd get nausea relief for exactly three hours, then feel gross for an entire hour. Notice the one thing I haven't mentioned: pain. I had been given a morphine clicker to use whenever I was in pain, but I never used it. Maybe I was afraid the morphine would give me more nausea, but I'd had it before with no such adverse effects, and to be honest, I just wasn't in pain anyway.

Once I got out of the horrible hot room and could sit up and think straight, I was no longer afraid. And I never did vomit from those 14 hours of anesthesia, which demonstrates what strong stomachs we have as people with emetophobia.

Today, I suffer from a chronic pain condition that stems from a car accident where I was stopped at a red light, and a big accident happened at the intersection when all the cars slid into mine. I got a sideways whiplash causing headaches that have lasted for decades. I take medications for the fatigue and pain, all of which list nausea and vomiting as possible side effects. I never cared. I have also had eight Covid-19 shots since the vaccines were first rolled out, and each and every time I get extreme body pain, plus a bunch of other symptoms. I know some people who died from Covid-19 and others who suffer from long-term Covid, so I persevere through it. Some of the shots made me feel nauseous, but I didn't care. I figured Covid-19 would be worse.

Chronic pain and fatigue mean that I can work at my computer for about four hours per day and no more. I have a bed with a mechanism that moves the head and feet up and cushions my aching body. I'm there now, with my laptop, as I wouldn't be able to write anywhere else for long hours. After I work the four hours each day, I try to do my limited exercise program of walking or going to the gym for about 45 minutes, and then I hit my bed. Usually, I have a package of ice for my neck and back. Thanks to the emetophobia community filling up my classes, workshops, and individual appointments, I was able to hire an assistant last year who works the other four hours a day that I should be working so I can continue to help as many people with emetophobia as I can before I flame out of this world for good.

I fear nothing to do with vomiting anymore. However, the surgery situation taught me that it's always there, that silly Golden Retriever waiting to lead me out of the building for no reason, so I can't get too cocky. I can still get a "jolt" if something comes at me sideways about vomiting. It might be someone suddenly vomiting on TV, or one of the grandkids coming to me to say their tummy hurts. I get the jolt, then inhale, and then it's gone.

One time, when I was in my late 50s, I experienced chest pain and was rushed to the ER by my youngest daughter. She's the one I was together with when we got norovirus. I was ushered quickly into a bed and hooked up to an IV and a bunch of heart monitors and ECG wires.

I looked at my daughter and with panic in my voice said to her, "I'm trapped here. What if I vomit?"

She said, "Mum, you're not afraid of that anymore."

"Oh yeah, right," I said, and the fear instantly dissolved.

You will not be 100 percent rid of your emetophobia after reading this book and working through the exercises. However, you can get there. Keep coming back to the exercises in this book again and again. If you feel like you've taken three steps forward and two back, remember that this is still progress. Whenever I've had patients or people I speak to online say they've slid "back to square one," it's never square one. You can easily figure out how far back you've slid by going to the videos—which ones do you think you can watch? You'll be surprised. Can you listen to the sounds? Then you're not anywhere near square one! What safety behaviors have you picked back up after giving them up? Give them up again. You can do it because you've done it before.

REVIEWING GOALS

Go back to Chapter One and review your SMART goals. Can you do any or all of them now? If you can, then give yourself a huge hug, go buy some balloons, and call the bagpiper. If not, journal about what obstacles are still in your way and make a plan to overcome them. Figure out what you can break down into smaller pieces so that they're easier to work on.

If goals are harder to accomplish, you'll want to try the following ideas:

1. Keep track of your progress:
   a. Decide on clear ways to measure your progress toward each SMART goal.
   b. Regularly check in to see how things are going.

2. Review your results:
   a. Make sure the goal is still clear and specific.
   b. Ask yourself if the goal was realistic, given your time and resources.
   c. See if the goal still makes sense within the bigger picture of your recovery.

  d. Check for any delays and how they've affected things.

3. Adjust as needed:
   a. Tweak your strategies if something isn't working.
   b. If circumstances change, modify the goal to keep it relevant.
   c. Get input from others to see what could be improved.

4. Find a therapist:
   a. If you can afford it, find a therapist who understands and has treated emetophobia, or at the very least specializes in OCD and anxiety disorders.
   b. Talk with your therapist about the work you've done so far, show them your plan from Chapter Nine, and ask them to help you stay accountable.
   c. If you haven't yet begun the exercises in this book, perhaps work through the book with your therapist. You may wish to suggest they buy their own copy or give them one as a gift.
   d. If you can't afford a therapist, especially one who specializes, see if you can get free counselling through any of the services provided in your community. Sometimes churches, synagogues, and mosques have clergypersons who will counsel you for free. They'll definitely need a copy of this book. But use your counselling time to talk about your progress and your feelings as you conquer the exercises and how they can help hold you accountable.

DEALING WITH SETBACKS

Once you feel as if you've made great progress and you're basically over the phobia, you will probably "go out into the world" and come across some sort of situation related to vomiting where you just "revert to type," as they say, meaning you behave exactly the same way as you did before you ever began your recovery journey. You will tend to beat yourself up about it. Refrain from that! This is completely normal, and it's your lizard brain's last kick at the cat, so to speak. To use my other metaphor, it's your poor misguided assistance dog trying once and for all to lead you out of the burning building without realizing that the fire was just a false alarm or a drill.

I remember shortly after I finished the group program with Dr. Philips I felt as if I was ahead of the game and could cope with one of my kids vomiting. My baby was about three or four months old. I cannot for the life of me remember what happened, but whatever it was I was very upset about it. Dr. Philips, who ran the program, was away on holiday but I was able to get an appointment with someone who worked with her. He reassured me that setbacks like this were normal and showed me a poster he'd made for a conference that was all about setbacks. He said, "See? They're so normal that I even have a whole poster about them." This made me feel much better and gave me hope and optimism to continue the journey.

When you inevitably fall back to the way you were all along, go sit out on your patio with a proverbial whiskey and a cigar and watch the sunset. (Canadians will need to sit by the fire for six months of the year.) Think about what happened, and how you could have behaved differently. This is not the same as just kicking yourself for behaving in the old manner. Close your eyes and imagine yourself handling the situation in a different way. Or write a story about it, again with yourself handling the situation and coping with all the feelings that may have arisen. Next time (and there will be one) you will tend to remember what you have thought about, and you will make better choices. This is all part of the journey toward wellness and healing.

MAINTAINING GAINS

Do your homework

As a CBT therapist, I give my patients and the people who are in my classes homework each week. I'm not talking about *that kind* of homework here. I'm talking about mental preparedness whenever you are going into a situation where you may be triggered. Let's say for a moment I'm about to take my grandson on an hour's drive to a nearby town. He gets carsick. My tendency might be to just "hope for the best" and throw the kid in the car. Or to give him motion sickness medicine or a bucket to hold on his lap, or both. In hoping for the best, I may be just in denial. Then if something happens and he's sick I will be shocked and horrified, and my anxiety might go through the roof.

If I "do my homework," however, I will mentally prepare myself for the worst to happen. Sure, I'll give him a garbage can to hold nearby, but I'll also prepare myself by saying something like: *Okay, so he'll probably vomit in the car. But he's old enough to vomit into the garbage can. He might warn me ahead of time, and I can pull the car over. I may get a jolt of electricity at the time, but then I'll just take a deep breath, and it will go away. I can cope with him vomiting. It will be a good experience for me and will help me to see that I'm farther along on this journey than I thought.*

"Doing my homework" is mental preparedness. It's being your own cheerleader before tough situations arise. Your closest support people may not even realize that a simple trip to the country would be something that would frighten you, so you're probably on your own with this type of preparation.

Diet and exercise

I'm not your mother, although I feel like it when I tell you to eat right and exercise. But I'll explain why. I have been reading posts from people with emetophobia for over 20 years online and have concluded that as a group, people with emetophobia have some of the worst diets of anyone in the country. I mean, their diets are really bad. Because many people with emetophobia only want to eat "safe" foods, those foods are often overprocessed, like granola bars, bread, dry crackers, soda pop, and even candy. The problem with this kind of diet is that while it sustains your life, it also puts your body into a state of fear for your survival, as many of the emetophobia "safe" foods have very little nutritional value. Robbed of protein, fiber, and vitamins, your body does all kinds of things that subtly make you feel sick. Many people with emetophobia, when they feel nauseous, revert to these types of foods.

Decide today to eat properly. Fresh fruits and vegetables, protein foods like meat, dairy, nuts, etc., and whole grains are not only good for you, but they're also relatively easy to digest, especially if your body has been craving the nutrients they provide for a long time. Try to begin tomorrow only eating foods listed in your country's food guide and nothing else. If you're feeling unwell you can drink clear fluids like fruit juice or broth made from meat or vegetables. I've made homemade jello with gelatin mixed into fruit juice to have when someone is ill or after a surgery. Clear juice popsicles are something else you can have when you are ill.

Many people with emetophobia avoid exercise altogether because they know that exercising to a state of exhaustion can cause nausea and vomiting. While this may be true, sitting around doing nothing physical is not the answer. Begin an exercise regime by just walking at a good clip for 30 minutes. After some time you can increase the time or the speed you walk at until perhaps you can try a light jog. If you can afford it, enroll at a gym, or better yet, find a sport you enjoy and join a team. Sports are relatively cheap compared to gym memberships. Walking, jogging, and even training for a marathon is free. An hour of exercise that gets your heart rate up (known as cardio or aerobic exercise) three times a week has been found in several scientific studies to lower anxiety levels in general, in some cases working as well as anti-anxiety medication.

Consistency

In order to stay in a state of recovery you must be consistent in working on your recovery. This means proper diet and exercise, reducing stress with mindfulness and self-care, avoiding all safety behaviors, and occasionally revisiting the concepts in this book. When you feel as though you are becoming anxious about vomiting again, and you're tempted to go back to your old ways of safety behaviors or avoidance, it's time to revisit the exposures. Think about which exposures you might be able to do with no anxiety, and which you might not want to do. Zero in on the ones you don't want to do! Perhaps it's that video of the guy on the news or the man on the plane. Perhaps it's those pictures of vomit. Whatever it is that you feel you'd rather not do, do it. Go back and look, because when you do it will always be easier than you've imagined.

Work ahead from there including the interoceptive exercises and then deepened extinction. Was there a time you volunteered in a school, hospital, or nursing home? Do you need to go back and do some more time there now? Sliding back, as I mentioned before, is normal. Sometimes it happens when you're under stress or have experienced trauma. It can also happen when other members of your family are under a great deal of stress or they experience trauma, whether or not they project their stress onto you. This is due to the fact that the pathway in your brain that went from your original triggers to a place of panic cannot be erased, removed, or destroyed. It is permanently there, even though it will deteriorate over time. Don't despair about it still being there, because if you've been working hard through this book, you have, by now, created an entire network of highways going from your triggers to many other places of peace, calm, and indifference. Those are also permanent.

Subjective units of distress (SUD), monthly average

Every once in a while it may help you to check in with yourself. Look back over the previous month and think of a number from 0 to 10, where 10 is the worst panic possible that would represent the *average amount* that you've been anxious. If I do it now, for myself, at this writing I'm going to give it a 3. As I think back, over the past month I was sick for half of it with H1N1 influenza. It didn't scare me (emetophobia-wise) but I made no money, and I had to reschedule patients, classes, and podcasts. My assistant also caught it so I had little help in the office. One grandchild melted down over a bully in their class and impending puberty. I went to Kelowna (a 40-minute flight) one weekend to watch my granddaughter curl, which was fun, but exhausting. Given these reflections, 3 isn't too bad a number. Almost always when I do this exercise now the number is 0 or 1. However, I've asked the question of patients many times and they've told me much higher numbers, often to their surprise. If your number is higher than 2 or 3, journal about what's happening in your life, noting all the stressors.

Keep reviewing goals

Keep those SMART goals handy, particularly if you feel you have been able to accomplish them all. Check back at least once a year that you're still able to do them. If not, it's time to think about why. Have you slipped back into safety behaviors, including avoidance? Has it been a stressful time for you or someone in your family? Then ask yourself which exercises in this book you think you can still do and which ones would be difficult. Start with the difficult ones and keep moving forward again until you can meet the goal once more.

Safety behaviors

The best advice I can give you is to catch yourself at the level of *wanting* to use a safety behavior before you just fall back into using one. For sure, if you catch yourself using one (or more) again, try to stop immediately. If you've fallen so far as to be using many or even all of them, print out one of those blank calendars and write in over *one* month the dates you're going to give them up again.

Avoidance behaviors can be very subtle. I've caught myself going downstairs to a different washroom when one of the kids is sick. And by caught myself, I mean literally, halfway down the stairs. I stopped and turned around, made my way back up and used the main washroom. I call this having a safety or avoidance behavior just "float by" with the beckoning "wanna come?" Resist at all costs. Stand firm in your recovery. This will be a life-long commitment.

Support person(s)

To help you stay in recovery, try to accumulate as many support persons as possible and tell them all the things you're likely to avoid, as well as give them a list of your safety behaviors. Asking for reassurance can be as simple as "Do you think this rice is okay to eat?" which most regular folks will just answer. They won't realize, and maybe you won't either, that they've fallen into your trap.

Self-esteem

Loving and caring for yourself is probably way overdue for you. I know that when I had emetophobia I spent a lot of time and self-talk in guilt and shame. I felt guilty for the way I treated my kids when they were sick, and I felt shame almost all the time for having such a "silly" phobia. I was always a wizard in school and felt pretty competent in my job, so I may have overcompensated for the shame and guilt I felt by trying to sound intelligent 100 percent of the time. People were intimidated by me and this helped keep my secret hidden. Once I recovered, I wasn't too sure what to do with all that guilt and shame, or any of the feelings I had around overcompensating for it.

Remember that your recovery will be slow and steady. You will have lots of time to figure out who you are without emetophobia because it won't happen suddenly. Slowly and surely, much like a dimmer switch being turned up rather than a "light bulb moment," you will become a different kind of person. You will be surprised at what the new you is like, how you will behave in the world, and how loving and empathetic you will have become. Don't leave yourself out of the love fest. You may have been beating yourself up for a long time, and there will be some scars on your psyche. But scar tissue is stronger than normal tissue, and you are stronger than you ever were and stronger than most people your age who have never had to go through anything challenging in their lives.

It can be helpful to keep a self-esteem journal to help you grow as a person without emetophobia. A sample is shown in Figure 10.2. Recording something you did well each and every day will not only help your self-esteem but will also keep you from overcompensating for your old self by boasting or making others feel bad. The more you love yourself, the more bandwidth you have to love others. Record your fun and positive experiences. You've had so many days with no fun, spending the whole day feeling sick or afraid or just miserable. Try to do something fun every single day: you're due.

I love counselling and teaching because I have fun helping people and passing on knowledge. Writing is fun for me, even as I watch the word count in the lower left corner of my screen tick slower than molasses. Every Friday night my daughter and I go to my sister's place a block away to have dinner and play Canasta with my sister and niece who live alone. I love my sister's cooking, and I love all the laughter around the table. I love the two nights a week that I go curling in the winter, and the two days I swim in the summer. I love TV dramas and movies, snuggled up with a purring cat. I love books and I alternate between literary fiction that's won the Governor General's Awards or a Pulitzer and a trashy thriller novel. I love checking Facebook every morning when I wake up and reading *The New York Times* and *The Globe and Mail*. I love 5.00-5.30 pm on Mondays and Wednesdays when my ballerina cum lawyer daughter calls me as she's driving home from work. I love playing ball and tug-of-war with my thinks-he's-a-lap-dog German Shepherd. I love going to church on Sunday mornings just to sing at the top of my lungs, and I have great fun connecting with old friends afterward as we drink tea in the lounge. Nothing I've said in this paragraph is normally thought of as fun, nor does it require going on vacation, and nor does it take any money. Be sure to have fun.

Date: ....

Monday	Something I did well today... .... Today I had fun when... .... I felt proud when... ....
Tuesday	Today I accomplished... .... I had a positive experience with... .... Something I did for someone... ....
Wednesday	I felt good about myself when... .... I was proud of someone else... .... Today was interesting because... ....
Thursday	Something I did well today... .... Today I had fun when... .... I felt proud when... ....

cont.

Friday	Today I accomplished... .... I had a positive experience with... .... Something I did for someone... ....
Saturday	I felt good about myself when... .... I was proud of someone else... .... Today was interesting because... ....
Sunday	Something I did well today... .... Today I had fun when... .... I felt proud when... ....

Figure 10.2. Self-esteem journal

Doing things for others is a wonderfully positive experience, which you may have neglected all those years you had emetophobia and your time was taken up being nauseous or afraid or both. You don't need to save the world. One small act of kindness can send ripples everywhere.

Medication, a final word

I am neither a physician nor a pharmacist, so there isn't much I can say about taking medication for emetophobia other than I know from experience with patients that it works. You or your doctor may have heard that meds don't work for specific phobias. This is true if you're afraid of clowns and normally only see clowns at a parade or on Hallowe'en. However, emetophobia is something that may plague you and make you anxious 365 days a year. It is also, as I have mentioned, related to OCD, which is highly treatable with medication. Therefore, it can be a lifesaver for people with emetophobia. It will not cure the problem, nor will it completely stop your anxious thoughts and feelings. However, it will take your anxiety down to a dull roar so you can function in life, as well as work on your phobia with ERP.

Many people who have emetophobia are afraid to take medication of any kind because they Google the side effects of the medication and find that nausea and vomiting are listed. I promise you that virtually every medication in the world lists nausea and vomiting as a side effect. This is because some people who take part in drug studies also get nauseous and/or vomit at the drop of a hat. If one of my girls took part in a drug study I can pretty much guarantee that she would vomit. That's because she vomits at the drop of a hat: too hot, too cold, new food, weird food, headache, fever, a cold, new drug, weird drug. You get the idea. I have spoken to literally thousands of people with emetophobia online and never yet have I talked with one who has vomited from any anti-anxiety drug such as an SSRI (selective serotonin reuptake inhibitor), SNRI (serotonin and norepinephrine reuptake inhibitor) or any of the newer types of these drugs. Many hundreds of people with emetophobia take these medications. You may find that they make you feel a bit "funny" or weird, and perhaps a little nauseous, but you won't be sick. If you're really worried, then work with your doctor and ask for a strong anti-emetic drug to take for a week or two while your body gets used to the drug. Your doctor can also start you on a very low dose and slowly increase it. Keep following your doctor's advice to increase the dosage until you actually feel better.

CAN EVERYONE RECOVER FROM EMETOPHOBIA?

I have met with and talked to hundreds of people with emetophobia over the years who were convinced that their emetophobia was so severe there was no way they could possibly overcome it. I only know of two or three for whom this seems to be true. So no, I don't think 100 percent of people can 100 percent recover. But 100 percent of people can benefit from therapy, exposure work, medication, and working through the exercises in a book like this one.

Some people may have a personality that is very low on courage and they may also experience depression so they're low on willingness to do the exercises. If this is you, it's not in any way your fault—you were probably born this way or had some sort of conditioning very early in childhood that meant you wound up not so courageous, and perhaps you also have a chemical problem in your brain as well. But considering you've read this far, I'm going to go ahead and assume you're still able to improve. People with zero courage don't buy books like this one, and they certainly don't read all the way to the end. Whatever small amount of courage you have, you can muster it. You can do hard things and you can cope with very difficult things including exposure therapy and yes, even vomiting. Moreover, you can cope with the amount of work that you need to do in order to recover.

Many, many people with emetophobia I've spoken to over the past 25 years say they have "tried CBT," "tried exposure therapy," or "tried everything," and thus concluded that they cannot be helped. I can't imagine how discouraging that must be, but I promise you that if this is you, you're probably wrong about it. If I'm talking on social media to someone who says they've "tried CBT," I ask them to elaborate. When they do, more often than not they've received cognitive therapy (the "C") without any behavioral therapy (the "B" and the "T"). Their therapist has gone to great lengths to give them worksheets where they write out their thoughts and the evidence for and against those thoughts, and so on. There is nothing wrong with this type of therapy, but for emetophobia, it just isn't enough on its own without exposure and response prevention, which is behavioral. I've also heard of therapists doing exposure work by telling their patients to start by going to YouTube and searching for vomit videos. This is about 50 rungs up the ladder, and I do not exaggerate. Many people share my experience with having their therapist tell them to start by sitting in an ER.

"Trying everything" can be quite extensive. There is a long list of types of therapies to try. Many who do hypnotherapy claim it can cure emetophobia, yet very few scientific studies have been done on hypnotherapy at this writing. One study I recall was just a case study of one patient. There are programs on the internet that claim to cure everyone of emetophobia and claim to be "evidence-based" when no evidence exists except what the creator of the program fabricated out of thin air. There are no internet police, and some countries don't even have regulations as to who can call themselves a psychotherapist.

Apart from the charlatans trying to exploit the desperate (those people with emetophobia), there are many legitimate therapy modalities whose practitioners probably believe they can help, even where no evidence exists. EMDR can be extremely helpful to process trauma, but again, only one case study exists for it "curing" emetophobia. Psychoanalysis might help if you can afford to see an analyst five days a week for five years, but there is no guarantee that it will. There are many more therapies, but the only actual evidence-based therapy to help emetophobia is ERP, or exposure and response prevention. A good CBT therapist will also do cognitive therapy with you to help you with your anxious thoughts, and most well-informed CBT therapists now incorporate ACT.

BEWARE OF YOUR FAMILY OF ORIGIN

Families have a state of balance among their members that we call *homeostasis*. The good is balanced with the bad. A fearful person is usually balanced with a chilled-out one. The "black sheep" who's always in trouble can be balanced out by literally every other member of the family being goodie-goodies. When a family is generally healthy (physically and/or mentally) but one person is not, family systems theorists call that person "the identified patient." This means that the whole family often has problems, but the problems of the others are diminished when one person seemingly takes all the stress.

If you are the identified patient in your family, the one with the problems, the one your parents worried and fretted about and were always trying to find help for, then you may need to beware of what happens when you overcome your emetophobia. If suddenly you're not the sick one, the needy one, the annoying one, the troublesome one, then where is all that negative energy in your family going to go? By getting well, you may have subconsciously upset the homeostasis of your family system. Unfortunately, when any living system's homeostasis is upset the system itself will subconsciously try to restore the system to its (old) homeostasis. So you may be inadvertently pushed back into being the identified patient.

Do mum and dad and big sis get together and say to one another

Hey, let's do everything we can so that Jane has emetophobia again? Of course not. Yet time and time again family systems researchers and therapists have seen it happen. Sometimes when the identified patient gets better, mum and dad have to start dealing with their own relationship that they've been neglecting for years while you took up all their time going to doctors and therapists. When big sis no longer feels a sense of superiority over you, or mum and dad start to focus on her problems, she may revolt. The whole family may revolt. Then your stress goes up and guess what rears its ugly head?

My first education was in marriage and family therapy. I did such counselling for years before going back to school and learning how to do CBT. So it's easy for me to tell you to "beware" but probably not helpful. All I can say is to *be aware* that these factors may be at play. Try not to get involved in family politics or the troubles of other members of your family, but stay in good emotional contact with them all. Remember to always put on your own oxygen mask first.

SUMMARY

- Recovery from emetophobia is a long road, and unlike overcoming a fear of puppies, for example, there's no puppy-like reward at the end—except for the freedom to live your life.
- Most people work diligently for one to two years before they're fully over emetophobia, but many stop before finishing because the last stretch is unstructured and requires more work.
- My emetophobia is 100 percent gone, though I sometimes still get a "jolt" when something takes me by surprise, but it passes in seconds.
- Recovery isn't instant—expect setbacks, but know that even if you slip, you'll never truly go back to the beginning.
- Reviewing your SMART goals will show how far you've come, and if you haven't met them all, break them into smaller steps and keep going.
- If you struggle, track your progress, review your results, adjust your approach, and consider working with a therapist

who understands emetophobia, or at least OCD and anxiety disorders.

- Setbacks are normal—when I had one, my therapist showed me a whole poster about how common they are.
- Before going into any situation that might trigger you, do your homework, meaning mentally prepare by imagining how you'll handle it.
- Eating proper meals with real nutrition will help boost your immune system and reduce your nausea over time. Regular physical activity helps reduce anxiety and should be part of your recovery plan.
- To stay recovered, stay consistent with exposures, avoid safety behaviors, and revisit exercises if you feel anxiety creeping back in.
- Medication can help lower your baseline anxiety so you can do the hard work of exposure therapy, and despite what Google says, you won't vomit from it.
- Many people say they've "tried everything," but most have either done cognitive therapy without exposures or exposures that were too extreme to start with.
- Your family might unknowingly try to push you back into the "sick" role because it disrupts the homeostasis of the family when you get better.

Appendix 1

Specific Phobia of Vomiting Inventory (SPOVI)

Please tick the box that best describes how your fear of vomiting has affected you over the past week, including today. A score of 10 or higher indicates emetophobia.

	Not at all (0)	**A little (1)**	**Often (2)**	**A lot (3)**	**All the time (4)**
1. I have been avoiding adults or children because of my fear of vomiting					
2. I have been avoiding objects that other people have touched because of my fear of vomiting					
3. I have been avoiding situations or activities because of my fear of vomiting					
4. I have been looking at others to see if they may be ill and vomiting					
5. I have escaped from situations because I am afraid I or others may vomit					
6. I have been restricting the amount or type of food I eat or alcohol I drink because of my fear of vomiting					

	Not at all (0)	A little (1)	Often (2)	A lot (3)	All the time (4)
7. I have been trying to avoid or control any thoughts or images about vomiting					
8. I have been feeling nauseous					
9. If I think I am going to vomit, I do something to try to stop myself from vomiting					
10. I have been trying to find reasons to explain why I feel nauseous					
11. I have been focused on whether I feel ill and may vomit, rather than on my surroundings					
12. I have been worrying about myself or others vomiting					
13. I have been thinking about how to stop myself or others from vomiting					
14. I have been seeking reassurance that I or others will not be ill and vomit					
Total					

Source: Veale, D., Ellison, N., Boschen, M. J., Costa, A., et al. (2012) 'Development of an inventory to measure specific phobia of vomiting (emetophobia).' *Cognitive Therapy and Research* 37, 3, 595–604. doi: 10.1007/s10608-012-9495-y.

Appendix 2

My Life with Emetophobia in Chronological Order

1960 My family moves to Bermuda when I am two years old.

1962 My brother dies in an accident.

1964 I tell my dad about my Obsessive-Compulsive Disorder (OCD) compulsions. He tells me they're "just habits" and to stop doing them, so I do.

1966 My family moves back to Canada.

1967 My sister gets married and moves away.

1968 My dad dies of cancer.

1968 Mother and I move to my dad's hometown of Kincardine, Ontario.

1974 I catch a virus at my sister's house and vomit several times. I was afraid beforehand, but don't recall being afraid once it started.

1976 I go to university in Waterloo, 150 km from home. I stop eating.

1977 I begin to eat, one bite at a time.

1979 I can eat normally again.

1980 I ask for a referral to a psychiatrist who I see for about two years. He wants to help me, but has no idea how.

1981 I get married.

1983 I take part in Dr. Clare Philips's Exposure and Response Prevention (ERP) group for vomiting phobia. By the end of the 10 sessions I am no longer concerned with feeling sick myself.

1983 My daughter is born. Fear of others vomiting escalates.

1985 Our third child is born and I return to university.

1990 I graduate with my Master's degree and am ordained as a minister. I avoid hospital ministry as much as possible. I run away, even from my own children.

1996 We take a car trip to Disneyland with the kids. The youngest vomits in the car and I totally lose it. Later that year I am diagnosed with cancer and undergo surgery and chemo.

1997 Further chemo and radiation. After being prescribed the wrong antibiotic I vomit for the first time in over 20 years. I was afraid for about an hour, then once I was sick I say to myself, "That was a big fat nothing!"

2000 I find an emetophobia discussion forum online and realize I'm not alone and there is a name for this phobia. A woman from the Netherlands puts up a web page with about 10 exposure pictures, beginning with eggs with faces drawn on and continuing to some pictures of people vomiting.

2001 After five years cancer-free I hold up my end of a bargain with God and try again to find a therapist to help me. I choose an excellent one (the 11th I have tried), although he knows nothing about emetophobia but is willing to learn. I have my husband print out the pictures from the online forum. I rent or buy movies on VHS that I know have vomiting scenes in them. I read about 20 books about the brain, anxiety, phobias, exposure therapy, Eye Movement Desensitization and Reprogramming (EMDR), etc. I am still not able to tolerate the sound, sight, or even knowledge of someone else feeling nauseous or being sick.

2002 After over 50 weeks in therapy and about 10 EMDR sessions, I decide to create my own gradual exposure system with the pictures and movie clips. I order a video called "Exposure to Vomit" from Ambassador Video, made by some psychologists in Sheffield, UK, who were trying to treat emetophobia. As a final step in this exposure therapy I volunteer as a chaplain at the local hospital for 14 days. I am able to volunteer on a medical ward, pediatrics, palliative care, and the Emergency Room (ER). I go in at 7 am for rounds and often stay until 9 pm. I am afraid, but believe I can cope with it now. Finally, someone vomits in my presence. I celebrate with my therapist at the end of the day.

2003–07 I take further study in counselling with a thought that one day I may be licensed as a psychotherapist. I finish my internship and residency while still working full-time as a minister.

2008 I crash from an unknown illness and go on medical leave. I am later diagnosed with severe fibromyalgia and put on four medications, which I take to this day.

2009 I have an elective double mastectomy reconstruction operation. The surgery takes 14 hours.

2010 I resign from ministry to begin my career as a therapist (online, on Skype). I put up one of the first websites for emetophobia information as well as a free resource website for other therapists treating emetophobia. I learn search engine optimization (SEO) to help spread the word, and eventually build my own websites and social media platforms, which are still active today. I contract norovirus along with my daughter at her basement suite in Edmonton, Alberta. I am not afraid at all.

2011–13 I take further study at the University of Alberta and finish my supervised hours for licensing (registration). I voluntarily take courses in Cognitive Behavioral Therapy (CBT) and OCD from Massachusetts General Hospital/Harvard University. I continue my own therapy for about 200 hours in total, processing childhood trauma and generally working toward being a more integrated, emotionally mature and wise person.

2013–18 My daughter starts a bakery 45 minutes from our home, and I scale back my career to help her five days a week. I see patients two days per week only. I do little work in SEO or social media during this time but my websites still have thousands of hits and backlinks. At one point my grandson vomits in my car but I am not afraid at all.

2020 I begin the podcast, *Emetophobia Help with Anna Christie*.

2022 I begin the Facebook group "Emetophobia No Panic," which, at this writing, has over 5000 members.

2024 Child psychologist Dr. David Russ and I publish the first book for therapists, entitled *Emetophobia: Understanding and Treating Fear of Vomiting in Children and Adults*.

Appendix 3

Three-Day Food Journal

Date: ....

MEAL	DAY 1	DAY 2	DAY 3 ....
BREAKFAST (first meal)			
SNACKS			
LUNCH (second meal)			
SNACKS			
DINNER (third meal)			
NOTES			

Appendix 4

Further Reading and Resources

EmetAction: Founded and run by academic researchers, this charity seeks donations for further research to be done on emetophobia. The website has general information about emetophobia as well as a blog: www.emetaction.org

WEBSITES

Emetophobia Help is my information website with a therapist list and other help for people with emetophobia: www.emetophobiahelp.org

Emetophobia Resources, a website from myself and Dr. David Russ, features resources for therapists treating emetophobia in adults and children: www.emetophobia.net

Turnaround is Dr. David Russ's website for helping children with anxiety: www.turnaroundanxiety.com

BOOKS

Harris, R. (2009) *ACT Made Simple: An Easy-to-Read Primer on Acceptance and Commitment Therapy*. New Harbinger Publications.

Harris, R. (2022) *The Happiness Trap: How to Stop Struggling and Start Living* (2nd edn). Shambhala.

Huebner, D. (2022) *Facing Mighty Fears About Throwing Up* (Dr. Dawn's Mini Books About Mighty Fears) (Illustrated edn). Jessica Kingsley Publishers.

Keyes, A. and Veale, D. (2021) *Free Yourself from Emetophobia: A CBT Self-Help Guide for a Fear of Vomiting*. Jessica Kingsley Publishers.

Lovitz, D. and Yusko, D. (2021) *Gag Reflections: Conquering a Fear of Vomit Through Exposure Therapy*. Toplight Books.

Roche, J. (2023) *Tummy Troubles: Gretchen Gets a GRIP on Her Fear of Throwing Up*. Magination Press.

Russ, D. (2022) *Emetophobia! The Ultimate Kids' Guide* (2nd edn). [E-book]. Skyline Publishing.

Thomas, J. J. and Eddy, K. T. (2019) *Cognitive-Behavioural Therapy for Avoidant/Restrictive Food Intake Disorder*. Cambridge University Press.

Watkins, S. (2018) *Scared to Be Sick: A Self-Help Workbook for Emetophobia*. Independent Publishing Network.

PODCASTS

Emetophobia Help with Anna Christie

The Emetophobia Podcast (Casey Vandemark)

Living Life with Emetophobia (Brooke & Maddie)

REVIEWS

My review of books and programs on emetophobia: https://emetophobiahelp.org/reviews

@emetophobiareview on Instagram and https://emetophobiareview.tumblr.com

Review movies and TV shows for vomit content.

BLOGS

Emetophobia Help: https://emetophobiahelp.org/blog

Emetophobia Resources: www.emetophobia.net

Stuff That Works: www.stuffthatworks.health/emetophobia

Turn Around Anxiety Blog: www.turnaroundanxiety.com/blog

David Veale: www.veale.co.uk/blog

SOCIAL MEDIA

Information and support groups can be found on virtually every social media platform. I have a presence on Facebook with a public information page "Emetophobia Help" and as founder of the private group "Emetophobia No Panic."

I post weekly to most other social media platforms such as Instagram, TikTok, X, YouTube, and Pinterest.

There are support groups on every platform, many of which are members asking for reassurance that they won't vomit or for information about safety behaviors. Patients should probably be cautioned away from these types of groups or asked to give them up when they give up other safety behaviors. Some pages on social media review movies and TV shows warn people with emetophobia away, but these can be turned around to use as exposures.

YOUTUBE CHANNELS

Dr David Veale: www.youtube.com/c/DrDavidVeale

Emetophobia Help with Anna Christie: www.youtube.com/user/EmetophobiaHelp

Anna and David's YouTube channel, ChristieRuss Emetophobia: www.youtube.com/@emetophobiaresources

Appendix 5

Glossary

A&E	Accident and Emergency (Emergency Room, ER)
ACT	Acceptance and Commitment Therapy
Anti-emetic	Anti-vomiting
ARFID	Avoidant/Restrictive Food Intake Disorder
CBT	Cognitive Behavioral Therapy
EMDR	Eye Movement Desensitization and Reprogramming
ER	Emergency Room (Accident and Emergency, A&E)
ERP	Exposure and Response Prevention
Gravol®	Dramamine® (anti-emetic over the counter, OTC)
Norovirus	"Stomach flu," "tummy bug," etc.
OCD	Obsessive-Compulsive Disorder
Ondansetron	Zofran
OTC	Over the counter
PMR	Progressive Muscle Relaxation
SNRI	Serotonin and norepinephrine reuptake inhibitor
SSRI	Selective serotonin reuptake inhibitor
Zofran	Ondansetron